KT-435-987

Nursing in Context

Policy, Politics, Profession

Michael Traynor
Middlesex University, London

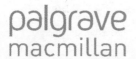

palgrave
macmillan

© Michael Traynor 2013

All rights reserved. No reproduction, copy or transmission of this
publication may be made without written permission.

No portion of this publication may be reproduced, copied or transmitted
save with written permission or in accordance with the provisions of the
Copyright, Designs and Patents Act 1988, or under the terms of any licence
permitting limited copying issued by the Copyright Licensing Agency,
Saffron House, 6–10 Kirby Street, London EC1N 8TS.

Any person who does any unauthorized act in relation to this publication
may be liable to criminal prosecution and civil claims for damages.

The author has asserted his right to be identified as the author of this
work in accordance with the Copyright, Designs and Patents Act 1988.

First published 2013 by
PALGRAVE MACMILLAN

Palgrave Macmillan in the UK is an imprint of Macmillan Publishers Limited,
registered in England, company number 785998, of Houndmills, Basingstoke,
Hampshire RG21 6XS.

Palgrave Macmillan in the US is a division of St Martin's Press LLC,
175 Fifth Avenue, New York, NY 10010.

Palgrave Macmillan is the global academic imprint of the above companies
and has companies and representatives throughout the world.

Palgrave® and Macmillan® are registered trademarks in the United States,
the United Kingdom, Europe and other countries.

ISBN 978–0–230–36873–6

This book is printed on paper suitable for recycling and made from fully
managed and sustained forest sources. Logging, pulping and manufacturing
processes are expected to conform to the environmental regulations of the
country of origin.

A catalogue record for this book is available from the British Library.

A catalog record for this book is available from the Library of Congress.

Contents

List of Tables and Figures

Tables

Figures

Acknowledgements

Hannah Cooke and Celia Davies helped with material that I drew on for Chapter 3, but it was their critical approach that I am most grateful for. Tanis Hand from the RCN provided information about healthcare support workers. I asked for a number and I got a whole history for use in Chapter 4. Thanks to Christine Beasley, Peter Carter and Jane Salvage for contributing their thoughts and experiences for Chapter 8. Jane Salvage also supported the idea of this book. Also, thanks to Nilam Mehta for her faultless transcription and Katie Stone for help with the statistics in Chapter 1. Finally thanks to my colleagues at Middlesex University for their ideas and discussions that gave rise to this book.

Introduction

On a good day on the hospital ward or in the clinic, things go reasonably well. Patients are given the time they need and are treated with respect. Procedures are explained fully, health professionals and patients are equal partners in care, ward leadership is empowering and teamwork is generally motivating. The multidisciplinary group of clinicians works well and each member contributes their own expertise ensuring the best decisions are made for patients. Senior managers put patients at the heart of their service. Dignity and safety are always paramount. Employment policies give staff the flexibility they need to run busy lives, and communication runs well both up and down the organisation. Government health policy is made, not in order to be seen to be making a mark, or to enact particular ideologies, but for the benefit of the users and to support providers of health care, taking careful note of those with experience of the service. Policy is implemented thoughtfully and evaluated objectively.

That's on a good day. Now let's add a few small but not unusual problems. Because of a financial problem, staffing levels are consistently a little lower than they should be, so patients get the minimum amount of time and attention they need for procedures to be done, and nursing staff are sometimes irritable. The ward manager lacks confidence, as she feels unsupported by her own manager and from time to time feels bullied by him. She is reluctant to tell him about problems on the ward, as action is rarely taken and she does not want a reputation as a troublemaker. Some members of the multidisciplinary team feel their professional opinions are only occasionally taken into account when decisions are made about patients, and some decisions made are unwise if not actually unsafe. They sometimes suspect that gender, race and class determine who gets a say in their meetings. The chief executive and the medical director do not get on well and have a constant battle over resources and clinical autonomy. The whole executive team feels under an almost impossible pressure to meet government targets and to reduce its expenditure by a significant amount, while a recent unexpected death threatens unwelcome media attention. Successive governments make a series of changes to the structure of the health service. Some are good, but others take up valuable energy on the part of health workers without delivering discernible improvements.

This book aims to tell the story of how nursing practice takes place in this real world of political forces and policy complexity. A look through the catalogues of most publishers' nursing textbooks reveals titles intended to prepare nurses for practice. There are books about anatomy and physiology, about drug calculations and those which set out to teach various skills. There are also books about professionalism and about autonomy and leadership. But too many turn a blind eye to the complexity of the context of practice and so fail in their aim to prepare nurses. Books that are naïve, simplified or idealistic can end up being part of the problem rather than part of the solution.

This book starts from the premise that it is only by acknowledging the complexity of nursing practice and its problems that we can analyse them in a way that sees them as examples of broader types of problem and so gain power over them and derive confidence and some therapeutic benefit into the bargain.

With this book, I invite you to take a possibly challenging, though always stimulating, and sometimes amusing, journey through eight chapters analysing the context in which contemporary nursing operates. I start by asking who today's nurses are and describing some of the profession's unusual history. I then discuss nurse training past and present, some of the tensions and advances and some of their unanticipated consequences. Chapter 3 presents some of the debates and issues with professional regulation and the troubled life of the Nursing and Midwifery Council and its predecessors. Chapter 4 looks at the professions 'next to' nursing – medicine and healthcare support work – and how tasks pass from one type of worker to another. Chapter 5 discusses the rise and establishment of the 'evidence-based' movement in health care. The final chapters discuss health policy and how a number of leaders of nursing influence policy. I round off the book on a future-orientated note by discussing how these leaders see the future of nursing in the United Kingdom.

Throughout I've included those familiar shaded boxes to suggest some thought experiments and other bizarre exercises you might want to try or to highlight some surprising statistic. I've used foot-notes extensively. This was a dangerous strategy because I've saved some of the best humour for them, even though I often skip these when reading in a hurry myself.

Evidence-Based Statement

Much of this book stems from research I have undertaken, most appearing here for the first time.

1

The Changing Face of Nursing: Who Are Today's Nurses?

The nursing profession – and what it means to be a nurse – is impossible to understand without some knowledge of its peculiar history. This first chapter sets out some of this history explaining the early moral obsession of the 19th-century culture in which modern nursing developed arguing that traces of this have remained and caused various problems. The chapter examines the changing demographic of those who join the profession, across its various areas, and compares it with similar information for medicine. It looks at changes to the ethos of professional work during the 20th and 21st centuries, changing views of authority over this period and mounting suspicion of the traditional professions. It discusses research into the motivation, over time, of those who have become nurses.

In this chapter you will find information about what the nursing workforce as a whole looks like today as well as its shape when 'modern' nursing was invented, in the mid-19th century. You will find out about why people choose nursing as a job and how nursing fits into various occupational classifications. But nursing has always had a lot to say about itself. Some of it has been, in my view, unhelpfully overblown. Today nursing is receiving a critical press, so this chapter is a chance to look at the unrealistic claims and set these beside the 'reality' of nursing.

When asked at the beginning of training (see section 'Why people choose, or decide not to choose, nursing as a career'), nearly all nurses, as well as midwives and healthcare support workers, say that they have chosen these occupations as careers because they want

4

to help people. Their training builds a range of technical capabilities and professional values upon this basic orientation. Yet out in the world of healthcare delivery, things occasionally go wrong and reports abound of nurses apparently failing to act in a caring way towards the patients in their charge. Given the context of high pressure, government targets for managers and falling staffing numbers, we should probably not be entirely surprised, though we can be disappointed and puzzled about causes. For reasons that I will go into in subsequent chapters, the profession has identified strongly with the powerful, if vague, notion of caring, so the fall from grace is especially hard. Having a realistic picture of what nursing is like may be a small but significant step to avoiding becoming dragged down into a cycle of disappointment, resentment and disconnection.

What are nurses and where did they come from?

There were just over 7 million nurses and midwives working worldwide in 2009[1] and about 0.63 million of those were employed in the United Kingdom, and 2.5 million in the United States. In 2003 the Royal College of Nursing of the United Kingdom published a definition of nursing:

> The use of clinical judgment in the provision of care to enable people to improve, maintain, or recover health, to cope with health problems, and to achieve the best possible quality of life, whatever their disease or disability, until death.
>
> Royal College of Nursing (2003)

Definitions of nursing, like those above, do not give much flavour of what it is to be 'out on the job'. The work itself is always more

---

[1] This was the most recent year for which data were available at the time of writing. The figure comes from a simple addition of highly incomplete WHO (World Health Organisation) Human Resources for Health data (http://www.who.int/research/en/) to which data from the United States Bureau of Labour Statistics (http://www.bls.gov) was added.

complex and messy than any definition. However, consider whether you would feel any different if your nurse tutors started their lectures like this:

> A nurse is privileged to be an integral part of God's design in the world of service ... The inspiration of Christian nursing is a history of love.
>
> Pearce, 1969, cited by Bradshaw (2009: 466)

There is no problem, of course, with religious interpretations of the world, but such pictures of nursing do require a level of buy-in on the part of the nurse and if you don't have it you are likely to feel excluded or just baffled. If you do have it, there are some troubling associations with notions of duty and self-sacrifice which I will discuss in Chapter 6. The quotation above is from Evelyn Pearce, once a prominent UK nurse and member of the General Nursing Council (one of the predecessors to today's Nursing and Midwifery Council – NMC). Some have seen her as one of the last apologists for Christian values in nursing and argued that after nursing's leaders abandoned this type of ethical claim, during the 1970s and 1980s, and market forces invaded health care (see Chapter 7), health systems witnessed a dramatic loss of public support for nurses. Ethicist Ann Bradshaw writes that without an ethic of duty nurses have lost 'the disposition to do the morally right thing even when no one is watching' (Bradshaw 2009: 466). So this is one kind of explanation for the question of why nursing may have fallen from grace with the public.

A few years after Evelyn Pearce made her statement, if you were reading nursing textbooks, you might have come across this statement about the importance of nursing:

> if we truly experience nursing as a kind of art–science, as a particular kind of flowing, synthesising, subjective–objective intersubjective dialogue, then nursing offers a unique path to human knowledge and it is our responsibility to try to describe and share it. (p. 102)

At its very base then, nursing is humanistic. It is, at once, man's expression of and his striving for survival and further development in community .... (p. 15)

Paterson and Zderard (1976)

You may need to read the above more than once. Explicitly Christian expectations of the nurse are absent here but they have been replaced with a new and equally grand project, humanism. Humanism with a focus on choice, rational abilities and the value of all people and the imperative that they determine their own destiny can be seen as clearly secular. But its concern with personal ethical training and the elements of ritual in various forms of humanism are familiarly 'religious'.[2] The point I am making is that many of nursing's leaders have made grand claims about the activity of nurses. Today's nurses may well be free from an overt Christian ethic of duty and service, but there are other powerful expectations at play and some say there remain vestiges of this religious ethic in the humanist aspiration to find personal fulfilment in being able to deliver high-quality care, to enable patients to achieve their full human potential and to have fulfilling and mutually respecting relationships with colleagues (Nelson 1995).[3]

Not wanting to dive into nursing's history too soon, I have so far avoided the F word – Florence – Nightingale. Although nursing has some ancient predecessors, its modern form, in most places in the world, developed from the work of British Victorian women, Florence Nightingale being the name that many people can remember. Its unique historical and cultural circumstances have stamped on the profession some characteristics that may have been useful

---

[2] See (http://en.wikipedia.org/wiki/Humanism) for a brief introduction to humanism and Sartre, J. P. (1957). Existentialism is a Humanism Written: Lecture given in 1946. *Existentialism from Dostoyevsky to Sartre W. Kaufman*. London, Meridian Books, Thames and Hudson for a position statement that has some resonances with the quotation from Paterson.

[3] What I am hinting at is that there is the danger of being set up to fail with such idealistic and possibly unrealistic aspirations.

in 1860 but in 2013, even in a faded form, seem puzzling or are unhelpful. In the 19th century, many of nursing's leaders presented the emerging profession in terms that would reassure male establishments, for example by emphasising the nurse's traits of 'obedience' and moral trainability. 'Do not let a nurse fancy herself a doctor' wrote Florence Nightingale in 1869.[4] Hierarchy, routine, helpfulness to doctors (a good preparation for marriage) and emphasis on rules of conduct become important in nurse training allowing nursing to be seen as preserving and developing 'womanly qualities' in its practitioners – unlike university education which many men of the time saw as threatening femininity and leading to ruin (Rafferty 1996). The bourgeois image of Victorian women was that their lives were largely devoted to domestic and family life. Cultural and Christian evangelical ideals of the period placed women on a pedestal of 'moral probity, motherhood and domestic orderliness' (Hudson 2011). As nursing's leaders came from 'substantial' (McGann 1992) middle-class backgrounds, it was predictable that the foundations of modern nursing would be ones that emphasised moral attributes.

However, as the 19th century wore on and during the 20th century, the basis for nursing's public legitimacy became largely, as in nearly all areas of public life, a story of increasing technicality and a waning language of moral qualities – hence the technical descriptions of nursing that nursing's organisations have set out. But societies do not hold one uniform value system. Just as the British industrial revolution of the 18th and 19th centuries was accompanied by a strongly critical romantic movement that recalled people to a humanity that was feared lost in the overwhelming rationality of the time,[5] so the 20th and 21st centuries have seen movements

---

[4] From a letter from Nightingale to Sir Henry Acland, MS Acland d.70 20 July 1869 f.10. Discussed by Anne Marie Rafferty in Rafferty, A. M. (1996). *The Politics of Nursing Knowledge.* London, Routledge. p. 44.
[5] The poetry of English poets Wordsworth (1770–1850) and Coleridge (1772–1834) promoted idyllic rural life and the realm of the non-rational as manifest in dreams, drug-induced states and myths.

that have promoted worldviews and values that are antithetical to rationality and science, for example various 'New Age' spiritualities and philosophical schools. I think the quotation from Paterson above can be understood as an attempt to link nursing work with a quasi-spiritual project and to promote a positive re-evaluation of nursing as not merely technical work. So, many of nursing's leaders today have been reluctant to let go of the religious roots that the profession has had, but the language of a 'religious' project has been replaced with secular terminology.

Who are today's nurses? How has the nursing workforce changed since the 19th century?

In the mid-19th century most waged work for women was in occupations associated with supposed female skills or characteristics; for example, domestic service was the single largest area of work of women in this period. As the industrial revolution developed, women became the major part of an entirely new workforce, particularly involved in textile production, partly because they were perceived as a flexible, cheap and adaptive workforce and, along with children, easier to recruit than men. However, there were considerable limits placed on women's public involvement. Married women could not 'engage in trade' (Levine 1863). Women were not admitted into the top universities (until well into the 20th century in some cases).[6] So in Victorian Britain nursing represented both a new opportunity for female employment and education (see Chapter 2) but also embodied sharp divisions in role and status in the workplace, notably between male doctors and female nurses. The social background from which nurses came changed little between the mid and late

---

[6] This may seem a world away but gender inequalities persist. Women's earnings remain below that of men, even when doing the same job. Women do two thirds of the world's work but earn only 10% of the world's income and own 1% of the world's property. Women are far more likely than men to be on the receiving end of sexual violence and, of course, dismissive or patronising attitudes. UNICEF (2007). Gender Equality – The Big Picture.

19th century. Although some matrons and superintendents were drawn from well-to-do families, most nurses were from relatively humble backgrounds. As religious sisterhoods declined in number and hospitals became more secularised, an explicitly religious orientation for nursing became increasingly irrelevant to most nurses who were simply 'ordinary women who needed to earn their living'

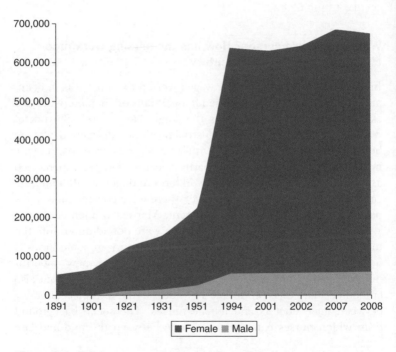

Figure 1.1 Total nurses registered in Great Britain by gender
Figures from 1891 are taken from Census of the Population for England and Wales, cited by Rafferty Rafferty, A. M. (1996). *The Politics of Nursing Knowledge*. London, Routledge; from 1901 to 1951 from Abel-Smith, B. (1960). *A History of the Nursing Profession*. London, Heinemann Educational. Figures from 1994 onwards are from NMC statistical analyses. Therefore, they are based on a mixture of national census data and registration data.

(Dingwall, Rafferty et al. 1988). The exalted claims made for nursing by some of its leaders fail to acknowledge this continuing and obvious reality.

In Great Britain the number of nurses has increased more than tenfold since the end of the 19th century to around 680,000 included in the register at the time of writing. The proportion of male nurses has also risen steadily (Fig. 1.1).

How old are today's nurses?

Those concerned with workforce planning for nursing have worried about the ageing profile of the profession. Figure 1.2, taken from NMC data,[7] shows that the nursing workforce in the United Kingdom is getting older. The proportion of under-30s has halved while that of the over-50s has increased from about one in every five of the workforce to just under one in three. This age breakdown also reflects the changing patterns of recruitment of student nurses with a decreasing proportion coming directly from school. Nursing shortages have tended to alternate with urgent recruitment drives in the United Kingdom, and the loss through retirement of a significant proportion of the workforce is likely to contribute towards a shortage at some point in the future.

Men in nursing

In 1891 approximately 54,000 people were employed as nurses, all but a little over 1% of them women. By 1901 this workforce had increased to 65,000 with a similar proportion of men. It was in 2002 that the proportion of men on the nursing register reached 10% for the first time.

In 2007, of 35,177 midwives registered with the NMC, 134 were men.

---

[7] The NMC has published yearly statistical analyses of its registration data. These are available from its website at http://www.nmc-uk.org.

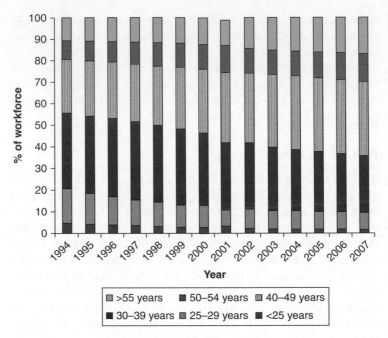

Figure 1.2 The changing age of the UK nursing workforce, 1994–2007

As we can see, men have been part of the nursing workforce since the late 19th century, though they make up only a very small proportion. They are not spread equally across the profession for a number of reasons. Men represent a little over 30% of mental health nurses but only approximately 8% of general nurses.[8] The well-discussed origin of present mental health services in historical asylums where men were traditionally employed gives a possible explanation. Also, and in common with most female-dominated

---

[8] This estimate is based on the last breakdown of gender by parts of the old form of registration provided by the NMC in 2004. After 2004 the register with 15 parts was replaced by a 3-part register – nurses, midwives and specialist community public health nurses.

occupations, men are disproportionately represented in management positions. In 2006 5% of the overall National Health Service (NHS) male workforce were men in management positions, compared to 2% for women, and senior managers made up 3% for males and 1% for females of the overall workforce.

Women at work

Female employment in the 1850s, 1860s and 1870s appears to have been higher than any recorded again until after the Second World War. In 1900 women's work still appears to reflect stereotypical female roles (see Table 1.1).

The proportion of women in work has risen. Today the numbers of men and women at work are almost equal, with UK men performing 12.8 million jobs and women 12.7 million, though almost half of these are part time. The evidence available suggests that by 2020 women will account for 80% of workforce growth. But, in addition to playing an increased role in the workplace, women continue to take disproportionate responsibility for home and family life compared to men (Green and Parker 2006). Often their choices about employment are determined, or rather limited, by the need for flexibility that springs from this. In the long term, nursing can be seen as flexible work, but opportunities for part-time or flexible

Table 1.1   Employment of women in 1900

Type of employment	Number of women employed
Domestic servants	1,740,800
Teachers	124,000
Nurses	68,000
Doctors	212
Architects	2

Data from http://www.historylearningsite.co.uk/women_in_1900.htm.

hours come at the price of lengthy training which is usually not flexible.

Women in nursing and medicine: What does it mean?

While nursing is clearly a predominantly female occupation, the stereotype of medicine as overwhelmingly male is becoming less accurate. Between approximately 2000 and 2010, the percentage of female hospital consultants and general practitioner principals increased from 19% and 30%, respectively, to 28% and 42% (Kilminster, Downes et al. 2007), and by the mid-2000s 60% of medical students were women causing some senior doctors concern that because of this the profession may start to lose some of its influence. How might that be? And if high numbers of women in an occupation are linked with low political influence and lower rewards, what does that say about nursing? This is how one journalist explained mechanisms of influence in medicine:

> The issue is about [doctors'] willingness to devote time, above and beyond their medical duties, to furthering the interests of the profession. That means eating dinners, attending meetings, sitting on committees – in short, networking. Men have been happy to give up their evenings for a chance to walk the corridors of power in the knowledge that their women have kept the home fires burning. Whether women will have the same confidence in their men – or the same desire to spend their spare time networking – is an important question.
>
> Laurance (2004)

This may be true but the association between female-dominated occupations and low rewards is more deep-seated than this explanation. Occupations that are seen to embody stereotypical female domestic activities, such as cleaning and childcare are amongst the lowest rewarded in many Western countries. It is as if the association of femininity with low occupational status can infect even traditionally powerful professions. Carol Black, President of the Royal College of Physicians, brought the issue to prominence in the mid-2000s, pointing out that in Russia, where medicine is almost entirely practised by women, the profession has very little influence, is ignored by the government and doctors have become 'just another part of the workforce' (BBC News Channel 2004). I think this phrase is central to the professional project – and I return to this idea throughout this book especially in Chapter 3.

The changing face of professional authority

As we have seen from this brief discussion on nursing in the 19th and early 20th centuries, Britain has changed hugely. It seems impossible to imagine today an economy and a culture where marriage meant the end of working life for women and it was expected that married women would retreat to the home and immerse themselves in dusting ornaments and Bex Bisselling[9] the carpets (before vacuum cleaners arrived), servicing husbands and looking after children. However, there are fewer and fewer people who have experienced life first-hand in 1940s and 1950s Britain. The 1960s saw major social and cultural changes. Virtually everything changed. Before then there was barely any pop music. Youth culture and the huge economic market that it presented were just about non-existent. Everybody on the radio had an accent that resembled that of the royal family. Vicars and doctors were noted members of their communities (in a positive sense). Few questioned the authority associated with a cluster of maleness, whiteness, establishment conservatism, expertise, moral uprightness and the (supposed) objectivity of science. This was the heyday of the professions, highly rewarded and highly influential. It is well accepted now that the decades since the 1960s have seen the steady erosion of unquestioned respect for conventional authority, including that once enjoyed by the professions. The four digits

---

[9] My mother had a Bex Bissell – and that was in the early 1960s.

'1968' have become signifiers for mass student protests, particularly in Paris, with a direct confrontation of authority.

Try this age and memory diversion: if you are in your 20s and reading this somewhere around the year 2014, you will have been born in the 1990s so will have no direct memory of the upheavals and excitements of the 1960s. However, an endless supply of late night television documentaries featuring psychedelic music, bizarre fashions and hairstyles from the 1960s and contemporary interviews with still cool (in a zombie-ish way) pop stars will make you feel like you were there. The point I am making is that it is easy to write that there has been a major loss of faith and respect for authority figures in most Western societies since the 1960s, but that statement won't mean the same to those who have never known anything different.

But by the end of the 1970s, the idealism of calls for freedom and of individuality had transformed into New Right politics, as the figures of Margaret Thatcher in Britain and Ronald Reagan in the United States set a direction and style of government that has never gone away, at least not so far. Part of the Thatcher project involved a direct challenge to collectives that were seen to stand in the way of the operation of a 'free-market' society of individuals looking to maximise their personal benefit through a series of economic choices. The trade unions were seen as one impediment to this vision, and the professions were another.

In the NHS, the Thatcher government saw professional self-interest as a, if not *the*, major problem. Powerful professional groups, particularly medicine, were, according to this viewpoint, self-serving elites, more concerned with building their own power base and gaining resources than practising a flexibility that would improve the service that patients experienced. NHS managers were simply administrators whose role was to support the work of doctors. I talk more about concepts of profession in Chapter 3 when discussing professional regulation and more about the policies adopted to reign in the power of doctors in Chapter 7. For now, I want to make the point that, whether we feel comfortable about it or not, the healthcare professions emerged from the 1980s and 1990s with a far more contested powerbase, less autonomy and more intrusion into their activities by agents of the state. I also want to mention that nursing, because it has been of less significance to policy makers, has often been caught up in the turbulence of policy initiatives aimed primarily at doctors.[10]

One feature of professional work that has become a battleground in health care since the mid-1980s has been 'autonomy' – the state-granted permission to make decisions about best treatment and to self-police members who fall below the standards of behaviour that the profession itself sets (see Chapter 3). The relationship between professions and the state is important because, in most cases, professions are granted particular protection under the law; for example, it is illegal to claim to be a doctor if you have not completed a particular, prescribed training (see Chapters 2 and 3). Autonomy took on such importance originally because the state itself unable to judge the performance of professionals was obliged to grant autonomy in return for assurances of quality and altruistic intentions (Light 1995). However, since the 1980s in many countries' health systems, techniques and procedures for monitoring clinical performance have become increasingly sophisticated and their results made public in the ratings given to whole hospitals or individual surgeons. Researchers (Harrison and Ahmad 2000; Timmermans and Berg 2003; Pinder, Petchey et al. 2005) have discussed the mechanisms and agencies that have developed in the United Kingdom and the United States since the 1980s by governments or insurance funders which record vast amounts of clinical and other data, set norms

---

[10] See Strong, P. and J. Robinson (1990) *The NHS – Under New Management*. Milton Keynes, Open University Press for a description of how nurses were affected during this period and for the compelling picture of nursing as an astronomical 'black hole', invisible to those outside it and caught up by the intense internal gravity of its own concerns.

for treatment and identify and perhaps punish deviations from these norms.[11]

After discussing the perceived status of professions within the healthcare system, in this last section I want to talk about nursing in terms of its 'official' occupational status and the reasons why people decide to enter the profession. First, we look at where different categorisations of occupations have placed nursing. Then we look at general influences on occupational aspiration, and finally we gather what's known about, why people choose, or decide not to choose, nursing as a career.

How various categorisations of occupations have placed nursing

The UK Office for National Statistics (see http://www.ons.gov.uk) publishes a Standard Occupational Classification (SOC) developed in 1990 and regularly revised as the patterns of UK occupations change (for example it reflects the rise of 'managerial' and computing jobs). The SOC classifies occupations into groups according to the concept of 'skill level' and 'skill specialisation'. This is based on the length of training and/or work experience that is recognised in each field of employment as being normally required to perform the activities related to that job 'in a competent and efficient manner'. The classification has four levels: the first corresponds to jobs that require only compulsory educational qualifications, and examples given are cleaners and catering assistants. The second level adds the requirement for a longer period of work-related training or work experience. Occupations classified at this level include machine

---

[11] At the time of writing, a useful and comprehensive list of characteristics of professions was available at http://en.wikipedia.org/wiki/Profession, though some of these are contentious or dated. One interesting characteristic mentioned is that professionals typically have individual clients. Although there are a small number of 'nurse entrepreneurs' (see Chapter 7) and independent midwives, this remains unusual in nursing as a whole. Nurses tend to rely on organisations for their employment.

operation, driving, caring occupations, retailing, and clerical and secretarial occupations. Level three occupations 'normally require a body of knowledge associated with a period of post-compulsory education but not normally to degree level', and these include technical and trades occupations. Finally, level four occupations feature the traditional 'professions' and usually require degree-level education or equivalent period of work experience. Nurses and midwives have their own group within this level.

However, a more fine-grained analysis is possible. In 2001 the Office for National Statistics replaced 'Social Class based on Occupation' (formerly the Registrar General's 'Social Class') and 'Socio-economic Groups' with a new 'Socio-Economic Classification' (NS-SEC) for all official statistics and surveys. In this classification nursing finds itself in 'lower professional and higher technical occupations' along with 'marketing and sales managers, technicians, midwives, radiographers, chiropodists, welfare and community workers, entertainers, surveyors, journalists, vocational and industrial trainers, ship's officers and immigration officers'.[12]

Some employment researchers have investigated the character of 'graduate' jobs. A nursing qualification may require years of study and extensive work experience but at present the number of graduates in the profession is small, though, of course rising. They describe nursing as one of a number of specialist niche occupations which require higher education skills and knowledge but which do not feature a large number of graduates within their ranks. They differentiate between 'traditional' graduate occupations (e.g. solicitors, doctors, lecturers, secondary school teachers) and 'modern' graduate occupations – the newer professions which graduates have been entering since the expansion of higher education in the 1960s (e.g. senior managers in large organisations, IT professionals, primary school teachers) with nursing fitting into the third 'niche professions' group (Elias and Purcell 2004: 4).

---

[12] See http://www.ons.gov.uk/ons/guide-method/classifications/current-standard-classifications/soc2010/soc2010-volume-3-ns-sec–rebased-on-soc2010–usermanual/index.html.

What class are you? One traditional view of occupational aspirations has been that class background has an influence, along with academic achievement, and gender, on career aspirations. A Youthscan survey undertaken in the mid-1980s, when the United Kingdom faced an economic downturn, found that children in families where the father was in a professional or managerial occupation were twice as likely to aspire to a similar occupation than children with working class fathers (Furlong 1993). A more recent study claims that: 'The historic and persistent link between British children's social class and their educational attainment is now well documented (Goldthorpe 2003; DES 2005), and indeed officially recognised (Strand 2007). There is little evidence that the class-based attainment gap is closing at primary level (DES 2005), and at secondary level the attainment gap in terms of class remains the widest of all the forms of social stratification (Strand 2007)' (Baars and ISC (University of Manchester) 2010: 2). Thinking about your own and your family's social mobility, would you agree with this?

Why people choose, or decide not to choose, nursing as a career

When asked, nurses and student nurses tend to say they chose nursing for its helping and people-centred character. When I asked just over 400 of the students who were just starting a nursing, midwifery or healthcare support worker course at our university in London in 2011 to rate the different motivations for taking up their course, I found that the most popular concerned caring for people and making a positive contribution to their lives. Reasons to do with career opportunities tended to come second (Fig. 1.3).[13] Other studies have found broadly the same, for example that altruistic motivations are most frequently named by first-year students undertaking non-medical health professional programmes but that the number of students identifying altruism and professional values and

---

[13] We used the same questions as the Nursing Research Unit at King's College London had used for their study of nursing careers, Robinson, S. and J. Bennett (2007). *Career Choices and Constraints: Influences on Direction and Retention in Nursing.* London, King's College London, Nursing Research Unit.

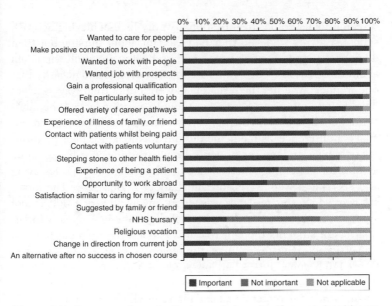

Figure 1.3 Reasons for starting nursing, midwifery or healthcare course in a London-based university, 2011 ($n = 410$)

rewards decreased over time (Miers, Rickaby et al. 2007). A large, longitudinal study undertaken by the Nursing Research Unit at Kings' College, London, included both diploma and graduate nurses from across the United Kingdom who had graduated 7 years previously. The main source of motivation and satisfaction that these nurses mentioned was to do with helping and the people-centred aspects of nursing work (Robinson and Bennett 2007). Outside the United Kingdom, a Norwegian study found that initially motives concerning human contact, helping others and job security were considered important by student nurses. However, towards the end of the bachelor course, there was more ambiguity in the helping motives (Rognstad and Aasland 2007). So it seems there can be some changes to motivation over time.

Finally, as light relief, what do we know about people who have considered nursing as a career but choose *not* to train? One piece of research focussed on this question. Twenty high-achieving Scottish school students who said they had thought about nursing but then decided to enter medicine or another healthcare profession talk about their reasons. Their views are so stereotypical and negative that one wonders whether the researchers went out of their way to select only brats to interview. For these students, nursing lacked the intellectual challenge of medicine, was routine by comparison, did not 'make a difference' as medicine did but was ideal for poor performing or female students, or students 'from a working class background' looking for something practical 'like hairdressing, joinery, bricklaying and secretarial work' (Neilson and Lauder 2008: 685). The larger study of which this research was a part, involving over 1,000 school students, appeared to bear out some of these opinions. Nearly three-quarters of students thought that it was not a requirement to go to university to qualify as a nurse, the majority of those who said they wanted to become nurses had low-grade performance in their exams and, according to the researcher, 'No pupils from social class 1 or 2 backgrounds (i.e. professional and managerial) chose to pursue nursing. Most pupils who had chosen to pursue nursing as a career came from social class 3 and 4' (Neilson 2008: 89–90). The conclusion that the researcher draws from this is that nursing does not do a good enough job of communicating the character and requirements of its work to school pupils.

Summary

In this chapter I've set out some of nursing's more grandiose claims about nursing work next to some statistics about the nursing workforce from its early days till today. I've talked a little about how the professions have been thought about, first in rather complimentary terms and then more critically. I finished by looking at classifications of occupations, including nursing, and closed with a summary of what is known about why people become nurses – and why they don't. On the way I have also mentioned the probably forgotten predecessor to the vacuum cleaner, the Bex Bissell.

2

Nursing Education: In and Out of the University

Students who read this book will be university students. This chapter summarises some of the struggles of nurses in the United Kingdom and around the world to raise the status of their training from an apprenticeship model with its associations with low status practical work to university level education with a strong intellectual and analytical component. The ethos of much higher education has changed particularly since the Second World War, and it has expanded, significantly, the entry of nursing from the early 1990s onwards contributing to that 'massification'. The chapter details an inevitable tension that remains between the intellectual and possibly critical aspirations of university education on the one hand and the needs of the workplace, especially the busy National Health Service (NHS), to have entrants who can 'hit the ground running' on the other. For health service managers, a certain amount of 'critical thinking' on the part of large groups of staff – like nurses – might aid efficiency but too much could be troublesome. The question arises, then, of where the nurse leaders of the future are prepared.

There is a strange double movement going on in public policy at the moment. On the one hand the UK NHS has agreed that the complexity of modern health care requires highly qualified nurses to do it justice – hence the agreement that from 2013 nurses needed a university degree to join the profession, a view supported by the Willis Commission (Willis 2012). On the other hand, we are witnessing the most significant cut in public sector spending for many decades. So those bodies who decide how many nurses their local

NHS requires and the managers in those NHS organisations who make decisions about recruitment are both cutting back on the wage bill. That means, putting it simply, fewer qualified nurses and more of the cheaper, flexible 'non-professional' workers like healthcare support workers and assistant practitioners. With nurse education it is often like this, as I show you in this chapter. The aspirations of the profession (at least of certain sections of it) seem to be at the mercy of the contingencies of other policy and economic events.

First, I set out some of the context of British higher education and then I focus on nurse education and show how the two, almost unimaginably, merged.

Higher education in Britain: Past and present

Let's go back to the beginning and look at university education in Britain around the time that nursing was being invented.

Before the mid-19th century higher education was only ever dreamt of as an activity for men. The first woman admitted to a university in Britain entered the University of London in 1878. The conservative regimes of Oxford and Cambridge, which had held a monopoly over English university education for seven centuries before the founding of the University of London in 1826,[1] did not formally award degrees to women until 1920 and 1947, respectively.[2]

But not only was it a purely male pastime, it was founded on and promoted a certain type of value. The following quotation from early in the 19th century gives a flavour.

---

[1] Oxford and Cambridge pre-date the oldest Scottish university, St. Andrews, founded in 1413.

[2] Anecdote: as a member of Senate of Cambridge University, I voted, in late 2011, for the university's new chancellor. Standing in the queue outside – unsurprisingly – Senate House, I started a conversation with an older woman. She described herself as a scientist and told me that she graduated from Cambridge in the late 1940s but with a diploma. Male students who had done exactly the same course as she had were awarded a degree. So this example of educational misogyny exists within living memory.

Without qualifying a man for any of the employments of life, it enriches and ennobles all. Without teaching him the peculiar business of any one office or calling, it enables him to act his part in each of them with better grace and more elevated carriage ... There must surely be a cultivation of the mind which is itself a good: a good of the highest order; without any immediate reference to bodily appetites, or wants of any kind ... and if Classical Education be regarded in this light there is none in which it will be found more faultless.

(Copleston, E. 1810) cited by Young (1992: 102–103)

In this defence of the Classics (Greek and Latin) against attack, the body and its appetites, employments and in fact anything too specific get short shrift compared to the promotion of a higher realm of the mind and vaguely spelt out personal qualities. It marks what Robert Young, who unearthed this quotation from Edward Coppleston, Professor of Poetry at Oxford, calls an example of the 'useless' knowledge that universities set out to teach – deliberately useless because the student at Oxford in the early 19th century would not require anything as vulgar as a specific employment. However, eventually the utilitarian values[3] promoted later in the century by figures such as John Stuart Mill and Jeremy Bentham mounted a more sustained critique of this outmoded argument, a critique and a debate that still echoes:

A sublime elevation versus a rational ground, useless Truth versus vulgar utility, quality of mind versus particular or practical

---

[3] Utilitarianism is an ethical approach claiming that the best or right course of action is the one that maximises the overall 'utility' that results, by whatever means necessary. In Victorian times its opponents thought it harshly mechanistic, and since then many have argued that it is internally inconsistent. It forms the basis of certain approaches to economic policy. Literary theorist Terry Eagleton wrote these eerily familiar words about the mid-19th century political ethos: '... a crassly philistine Utilitarianism is rapidly becoming the dominant ideology of the industrial middle class, fetishising fact, reducing human relations to market exchanges and dismissing art as unprofitable ornamentation'. Eagleton, T. (1983). *Literary Theory: An Introduction*. Oxford, Blackwell, p. 19.

use: such were the terms of the debate which, in spite of local variations, has remained the basis of discussions of university education from that day to this.

Young (1992: 103)

Coppleston's ideas were possibly a little archaic even when he expressed them, and are a specific defence of the teaching of Classics but today some of his points translate into what we might call Liberal educational ideals. Here's a useful definition:

Ideally, a liberal education produces persons who are open-minded and free from provincialism, dogma, preconception, and ideology; conscious of their opinions and judgments; reflective of their actions; and aware of their place in the social and natural worlds....Liberally educated people are skeptical of their own traditions; they are trained to think for themselves rather than defer to authority.

Wikipedia Contributors (2011)

So, before we continue with this line of argument, let's quickly ask what this might mean for nursing. One research team claimed to have noticed a difference between how nurses and doctors conceived of professionalism (Walby and Greenwell 1994). They wrote: 'the nursing notion [of professional activity] was one of technicality, of pinning down exactly what was to be done and the training and staff needed to do it to agreed standards... nurses often saw professionalism as being a rule-governed process, intimately tied in with checking and monitoring' (Walby and Greenwell 1994: 61). They claimed that the doctors in their study undertaken in the NHS in the early 1990s appeared to hold a view of the professional as 'an educated person able to respond to individual problems in undetermined, innovative yet trustworthy ways' (p. 61). Their conclusion clearly covers over a degree of variation, but the point they make is something like this: professional work can be conceived of and organised as a number of specific tasks, for which specific, defined and testable competencies and 'skills' are required. Or it can be understood as a field of activity within which the well-educated professional makes critical judgements. One of the liberal arguments for degree-level nursing entry would be that health care is now so complex and unpredictable that it is impossible to think of preparation as simply learning a large amount of information and the skills that should be applied to a set of activities and circumstances. It is far better, the argument goes, to equip nurses with broader abilities and general approaches so that they can, in the words above, 'think for themselves rather than defer to authority', even the authority of textbooks, teachers and managers. But does the health service really want this? We will return to that question later.

Changes in UK higher education since the Second World War

Let's fast-forward through the 19th century, the First World War (1914–1918) and the Second (1939–1945). By now the expectation of universities has changed significantly, from an independent, at times critical, elitist system expected to produce the country's leaders, to a centrally controlled mechanism for serving the needs of the country's growing post-war economy by producing a suitably prepared workforce in appropriate numbers. In the 'opportunity' culture of the 1950s and under the influence of a growing industrial sector, British university education came to be seen more as 'a means of employment than as a civilising community' (Becher and Kogan 1992: 28). The elitist view that universities should provide the next generation of scholars and leaders was beginning to crumble under a growing pressure for employment relevance. By the 1950s, the numbers of school leavers entering higher education in Great Britain had risen from 1 in 60 before the war, to 1 in 31 (Becher and Kogan 1992). In the early 1960s, about 1 in 20 young people were going into higher education (BBC News 2010). Today about one in five school leavers goes on to higher education with female students overrepresented.

Women students obtained 23% of all first degrees in the academic year beginning 1922. By 1980 this had risen to 37% and in 1993, 45%. Thus the trend over the last century has been towards equalisation. In the early part of the 20th century the most popular full-time university faculty, for both men and women, was the Arts. In 1996 the most popular faculties were engineering and technology for men, and social studies for women.

A Century of Change: Trends in UK Statistics Since 1900 (1999)

British culture seems never to miss an opportunity to act out its class structure. In the 1960s, to accommodate the rising demand and increasingly vocational character of courses required, the government introduced a two-level approach to higher education. It consisted of on the one hand locally controlled technical colleges, colleges of education and polytechnics and on the other the traditional universities. It was an explicitly 'dual system' with each sector making its own distinctive contribution. The universities were to remain national in their recruitment, while colleges and polytechnics were to be locally funded and regionally focussed. However, in other ways, the difference was artificial and over the years the polytechnics increasingly took up the universities' traditional aspirations while universities moved towards 'meeting identifiable market needs' previously largely addressed by the public sector colleges (Becher and Kogan 1992: 31).

Higher education expanded cautiously during the 1970s, but during the 1980s and early part of the 1990s the government encouraged rapid growth. In 1988 the polytechnics were removed from local authority control, and shortly afterwards, as a result of the Further and Higher Education Act of 1992, the binary line separating universities and polytechnics was abolished and polytechnics were given the title of university. Heads of the former polytechnics had the task of coming up with ingenious names for their institution if the established university in their city already had the city's name. The encouragement of university expansion caused a drastic change in recruitment patterns. Successful applicants were now more likely to have lower A-level scores or non-traditional qualifications. The system as a whole could no longer be said to be elitist.

This rapid expansion, or 'massification', of higher education, however, led to a greater variety between and within institutions. New, and often vocationally orientated subjects, such as nursing, were added to the university curriculum. They may have been more difficult to absorb than traditionally high status subjects such as law and medicine, partly because of the relatively low occupational status associated with them, but they represented too good a business opportunity for university managers to miss. Nursing put the 'mass' into massification. The separation between an education based on knowledge-gathering and skills acquisition on the one hand, and on the other an initiation into an intellectual or professional culture has become harder to sustain in the changing climate of the last 20 years.

In July 1997, The National Committee of Inquiry into Higher Education, chaired by Sir Ron Dearing, reported on its investigations into the higher education sector across the United Kingdom. It made a significant restatement of a utilitarian and largely market-driven view of higher education that has remained and intensified since its publication. This was the first major review of higher education in the United Kingdom for 30 years. The committee's wide-ranging remit was to 'make recommendations on how the purposes, shape, structure, size and funding of higher education, including support of students, should develop to meet the needs of the United Kingdom over the next 20 years . . .' (National Committee of Inquiry into Higher Education 1997 para. 1). The review was commissioned by an outgoing Conservative administration and reported to the new Labour government. The initial publicity that the report gained centred around one of its 93 recommendations that students should contribute towards the cost of their tuition. Already it is hard to believe that at one time no home student paid tuition fees. One response in *Nursing Standard* asked whether the prospect of tuition fees would raise a barrier to nurse recruitment (Allen 1997); however, the government made funding of nursing students a special case (Nursing Standard News 1997). Nurses undertaking degree courses were to have tuition fees paid by the Higher Education

Funding Councils and, in addition, have access to bursaries. The majority of student nurses, those completing diploma courses, would continue to receive funding through the NHS. The same arguments, those of a 'crisis' in staffing levels, were offered by those urging that medical students too should be exempt from university tuition fees (Brown 1997). A matter of weeks later, the government announced that all pre-registration nurse training, diploma and degree level courses alike, would be funded by the NHS via the decentralised Education and Training Consortia.

The Dearing report presented a picture of higher education in economic and market terms, part of the armoury the nation would need to defend against economic competition from ambitious Far Eastern economies. Education was a commodity that individuals chose to invest in for a return. But the report attempted the difficult balancing act of promoting the role of universities as supplying this competitive workforce while simultaneously acting as a site for the transmission of society's values and for developing 'individual fulfil-ment'. There is an assumption that the critically minded products of universities, including nursing graduates, will be just critical enough to help their managers' organisations to work more efficiently but not so critical that they ask questions about why we need that industry or whether things could fundamentally change. In support of this analysis, it is common to hear managers in many sectors say that they want 'competent' new workers who can 'hit the ground running' and complaints abound that graduates, including nurses, are not fit for purpose with basic skills. In universities, however, variants of the liberal educational ideals set out above are widely expressed along with a view that universities should be critics of the state and not merely a cog in its economic machinery. So there is a tension, and I go on to discuss the particular way that this is played out in nurse education which has to fulfil considerable external requirements.

Nurse education

As I discussed in the previous chapter, nursing's history has involved both its promotion as a fundamentally ethical activity and as one based on technical expertise and autonomy of practice, with established professional characteristics as a model. I argued that both ways of understanding nursing work could be useful but both have fuelled a series of idealised fantasies that end up confusing and demoralising actual nurses.

The first mid-19th century nurse training was 'character' training, couched in an ethical language. This was for a number of reasons. First, Florence Nightingale and others at this time saw themselves as reformers of nursing. 'Nursing' before the reformers was done by independent women who worked in the homes of the sick, providing a range of services including basic tasks and laying out of the dead (Rafferty 1996). Accurately or otherwise, those promoting nursing reforms, supported by the medical establishment, presented this unsupervised group of women workers as morally lax and quite possibly drunk on the job. Drunkenness for the Victorian establishment held the same horrors that looting and drug taking does today. Drunkenness and poverty were seen as serious social threats to the paranoid Victorian middle class. Emphasising temperance in alcohol intake and in character was an ideal way of distancing the new nursing from its predecessors and was also a way of promoting these qualities among the poorer classes with whom nurses would come in contact. Second, as we have already seen, for many at this time education was understood as a fundamentally character-centred process, so Nightingale's emphasis on this was not unusual. Third, work in hospitals, rather than in the multitude of homes of individual clients, required reliability and discipline in order to fit into its production processes as well as self-control in the face of possible repulsion, as it still does today. Finally, nursing reforms were unlikely to get far if the male establishment on which it relied for support was unsettled by strident feminist talk, so docility and obedience were emphasised as central to training. So a number of pragmatic forces shaped the foundations of nurse training, and the emphasis on obedience and discipline within the convent-like walls of the hospital and nursing home lingered well into the 20th century.

Unfortunately, although there are some similarities between Nightingale's moral training and the character transformations said to accompany a liberal education, there is one major feature absent in the model attributed to Nightingale and that is criticality. The succinct definition of liberally educated people as sceptical of their own traditions and trained to think for themselves rather than defer to authority would make many nurse tutors of the past turn in their graves. In fact many have blamed the view of nursing as an essentially moral activity for a culture of anti-intellectualism that some see as plaguing the profession ever since (Johnson 1974). The idea of nurse training occurring in universities was so far from the minds of the nurse reformers who followed Nightingale that it was never part of their campaign to promote the profession. They did not involve nursing, for example, in the debates that were raging at the turn of the 19th century about opening the universities of Oxford and Cambridge to women, discussed earlier. However, some of the reformers were influenced by nurse leaders in North America where the profession was working for, and succeeded in gaining, entry into universities and colleges. It was the investment of the American philanthropic Rockefeller Foundation in British nursing that opened the way to the founding of one of the first university departments of nursing in the late 1950s.

In 1959 the first university diploma in community nursing was established at the University of Manchester, and in the following year the University of Edinburgh offered the first undergraduate pre-registration programme for nursing. The first Bachelor of Nursing degree course was established in 1969 also at the University of Manchester.[4]

Basic nurse education had been delivered in over 600 schools of nursing in England in the early 1970s but a series of amalgamations left less than 200 by the mid-1980s. Yet the period also witnessed the proliferation of educational courses for nurses, including degree courses, which were taught and awarded in association with a number of colleges and universities.

---

[4] By 1994, 25 pre-registration nursing degree programmes existed in UK universities. Royal College of Nursing (1996). *A Principled Approach To Nurse Education. The Rationale. A Document for Discussion*. London, RCN.

A popular nursing text book from the 1930s shows diagrams of
different designs of toilet, drainage and heating systems in the same
detail as the systems of the body. It also gives advice about the most
hygienic ways to dress as well as how to keep a half-filled milk bottle
free from contamination by means of a tumbler (Modern Mental Nursing
by Douglas Hay Scott and colleagues published by Caxton).

Briggs and Project 2000

In 1972, the Committee on Nursing chaired by historian Asa Briggs
(Committee on Nursing 1972) considered nursing in the NHS
and criticised its state of neglect. The committee strongly recommended both a restructuring of the profession's regulatory bodies
(see Chapter 3) and a radical reform of nurse education. The report
concluded that existing training was spread too thinly across nearly
655 schools of nursing in England and Wales and 62 in Scotland.
It featured specialisation e.g. as children's or mental handicap nurses
too early on, making workforce planning difficult. Somewhat out of
tune with today's thinking, the committee rejected the RCN's call
for an increase in the qualifications required of recruits to nurse
training. Instead it wanted to place more emphasis on motivation
than on formal academic achievement. The report recommended
reducing the age of entry to training from 18 to 17 and changing the
structure of education involving two 18-month parts. It also recommended setting up a new body to oversee education and registration,
the United Kingdom Central Council for Nursing, Midwifery and
Health Visiting, the UKCC.

So in the mid-1980s, the UKCC started work on devising a
major reform of nursing education in the United Kingdom. That
reform became known as Project 2000. The first aim was to change
the nature of nurse education, from a system which was largely
driven by the requirement to meet the NHS workforce needs with
its large contribution of student labour, to one that would expose
its students, as well as those who educated them, to the hopefully beneficial effects of mainstream higher education. However,

action on this reform was not taken until more than a decade after the original recommendation. The UKCC's document argued that change was urgent if nursing was to be seen as a vibrant profession (United Kingdom Central Council for Nursing Midwifery and Health Visiting 1986).

As with the movement behind more recent reforms, the report drew attention to the impact on healthcare needs of a complex set of social changes. A further factor marshalled as supporting change was the so-called demographic 'time bomb', a reducing pool of 18-year-olds from which nursing had traditionally recruited combined with an overall ageing population. Of course, as the symbolic interactionists[5] tell us, we don't tend to act towards things and events in themselves but towards the meanings we invest in them. Nurse training before the university was often described as 'an apprenticeship model'. Whatever variety of actual practices is included by that term, the association was one of how trade skills, plumbing for example, were transmitted from experienced tradesmen to their 'apprentices'. Alongside all the other arguments for university-based education, many in nursing felt that the association with trades did not help the overall status of the profession.

In a profession with deep historical divisions over the question of intellectual education and character qualities, an unusual moment of consensus was emerging. Educators felt the pressure of an ever-growing curriculum, while managers of the service were faced with the challenge of the increasing complexity of hospital work and a new emphasis on health care provided in the community. Wastage rates were also high; the service lost 30,000 nurses each year and a high proportion of student nurses left during training (Davies 1995). Of those who started nurse training in England and Wales, only 65% successfully reached the register (United Kingdom Central Council for Nursing Midwifery and Health Visiting 1986). The Project committee held over 40 formal meetings with nurses in the four

---

[5] Symbolic interactionism is a theory within sociology first developed in the late 1960s. See Blumer, H. G. (1969). *Collective Behavior. Principles of Sociology*. A. McClung Lee. New York, Barnes and Noble Books, 65–121.

countries of the United Kingdom and many more informal consultations. These meetings and other responses convinced the committee of a 'depth of frustration and dissatisfaction' within the profession at large.

In response, Project 2000 recommended an educational structure based on a year's common foundation programme followed by a number of specialist branches: adult, children, mental health and learning disability. Enrolled nurse (EN) or so-called second level, or more practical training introduced to help bolster nursing recruitment during the post–Second World War years, which was shorter than that for registration, was to end but opportunities for retraining with this level of qualification were to be provided. Students were, for the first time, to enjoy supernumerary status and to be funded by higher education grants rather than receive a wage from health authorities. The idea behind both of these changes was that observation and learning would be far more likely to occur than if students were counted into workforce numbers and under pressure to 'get through the work'. It is not clear though how far a genuine change in ethos has ever occurred where highly pressurised nursing staff bend over backwards to facilitate the learning and critical reflection of students. The new system was expected to reduce wastage considerably, and 64–70% of the nursing workforce was envisaged as being made up of trained nurses.

The scheme, however, ran into problems. The government expressed commitment but declared its cost to be unacceptably high. It also disagreed about the ending of EN training and argued that attention needed to be given to the recruitment of an untrained, support workforce. Funding was to allow only half the former students to be replaced with qualified nurses. Regional Health Authorities, which at the time were part of the NHS structure with a largely strategic role, were asked to put forward submissions for schemes from institutions in a very short time scale and, in the first year, only 13 of the 23 submissions were approved. By 1992, 4 years after the scheme's acceptance, four out of five nursing students were Project 2000 students while 17 colleges were still running the old courses (Davies 1995).

A National Audit Office enquiry into the Project's implementation identified the problems that the concurrent move to reduce public expenditure had caused it (National Audit Office 1992), while nurses themselves complained that the speed and confusion surrounding the implementation had affected recruitment.

Unanticipated problems

However, a further unanticipated and more far-reaching problem faced the scheme in the shape of the proposals to radically reform the NHS into an 'internal market' which were first announced in January 1989 (Department of Health 1989). As a result, colleges and schools of nursing were required to contract with local healthcare providers to meet the staffing and skill mix needs that the providers themselves identified. In addition the National Vocational Qualifications (NVQ) scheme was to be extended to allow an increased number of support workers to be trained and employed. Nursing's educational aspiration was compromised at the very moment that it could have been realised:

> The Project 2000 vision of a clearly demarcated and separate educational budget, managed by schools themselves, was being thoroughly overtaken by the new contract culture of the NHS.
>
> Davies (1995: 123)

Nurse education began its move from NHS colleges of nursing into the higher education sector in 1991. An unforeseen implication of the 1990 NHS and Community Care Act was that schools of nursing no longer had a place within NHS provider trusts. For definitions and discussion of what exactly 'provider trusts' were, see Chapter 7. Some commentators at the time suggested that the move of nursing into higher education occurred for a number of reasons, some of them have little to do with educational idealism:

> A cynic might argue that the merger of colleges of nursing with university departments is occurring because the desire of health

authorities in the U K to dispense with the inconvenience of nurse training coincides with the willingness of the universities to take over a promising business opportunity.

Draper (1995: 214)

Others noted, in a similar vein, that with some of these mergers, 'the higher education partner achieves an instant increase in numbers – of as much as 30% – and adds an additional school, or faculty, to its academic menu' (Fletcher 1995: 35).

As a further unanticipated development, the restructuring of higher education in the United Kingdom after the Further and Higher Education Act of 1992, detailed above, meant that, apart from those already in the traditional university sector, nursing's teaching workforce experienced a major upheaval in terms of culture and infrastructure. Nurse tutors who had been dragged from schools of nursing into polytechnics had barely time to take a breath before finding themselves working in universities alongside more established career academics. The culture of many schools of nursing had owed more to the junior school than to higher education with a focus on discipline and their tutors uncomfortable with students who asked questions. The thinking was that the relocation to universities would cause a new more intellectual culture to seep into nurse education – and educators. For the most part this has to be true; however, the combination of large student cohorts, a curriculum fundamentally set by outside bodies and a certain lack of confidence among tutors new to university teaching can thwart some of the university's ambitions for high level education.

New knowledge or old? Try to imagine a tension that might have emerged in those early days between the idea of the university as generator of new knowledge (through the research undertaken there) and of nurse training as the promulgation of a textbook of already existing facts to be learnt, remembered and put into action (how the heart works, how to do a bed bath). Perhaps it will always require a certain force of will to reconcile this tension between the health service's desire for safe and respectful workers (and for a supply of people who can train them to be these workers), and the open debate and experiment that, on a good day, characterises the university.

The 2011 changes: Degrees and controversy

The same array of changes – to society and to health care – named in support of Project 2000 have been, 20 years later, marshalled as the impetus for the most recent changes to nurse education. Cultural diversity, health inequalities, an aging population, increased expectations from patients and their families, complex technology, the pace of patient throughput and the often repeated 'need for a flexible workforce' are all cited as the context for a need to change nursing careers and nurse education in the document Modernising Nursing Careers released in 2006 by the Department of Health and Chief Nursing Officers of the United Kingdom (Department of Health and CNO's Office 2006). This publication sets out a range of aspirations for nursing, and many are so general that it is hard to disagree with the overall spirit behind them. Some ideas, however, are so radical that it is hard to imagine them being proposed for a professional group seen to be less 'flexible' than nursing. While medicine world-wide remains largely organised around bodily systems, *Modernising Nursing Careers* proposes that nursing roles and careers are based around patient pathways and needs. Some of the recent changes to nurse education in England reflect the drive for 'flexibility'. Other drivers to do with the supply of nurses include the desire to maintain recruitment, particularly in the face of an ageing nursing workforce. Degrees are seen to be a more attractive currency than diplomas especially for bright school leavers, and particularly against the background of what some have seen as 'qualifications inflation', i.e. that yesterday's diploma is today's degree; today's degree is tomorrow's master's degree and so on.

Nurse education is extremely highly specified by bodies external to those which provide it. The NMC regularly sets out what it considers are the adequate standards required for education and competence for registration as a nurse or midwife. The most recent set of these standards was published in 2010 (Nursing and Midwifery Council 2010). The NMC itself is obliged to incorporate directives from the European Parliament regarding the recognition of professional qualifications within Europe. This includes specific requirements on programme length, content and ratio of theory to practice, and the nature of practice learning and range of experience. The whole course, for example, must be no shorter than 4,600 hours, split equally between theoretical teaching and practical work experience. The NMC's document sets out requirements for the timing of assessments and the character of the final judgement of competence to join the register. The universities that provide such courses have themselves to meet the NMC's strict requirements. The NMC bases its notion of ability to join the register around the concept of 'competence'. This is not seen as technical ability to complete a task alone but is described in terms of a global readiness involving a combination of skills, knowledge and attitudes, values and technical abilities. The notion of education and particularly vocational training based on competence was promoted in the United Kingdom and other industrialised countries during the 1980s and 1990s as part of the movement I've already discussed to make education, including higher education, more relevant to what employers say they want from their employees. The movement and its underlying concepts have been critiqued on a number of grounds, among them their unsuitability for higher education because a model aiming to bring individuals to a preset standard does not square with a view of education as constantly questioning such standards. Others have criticised the effect of the drive for behaviours that can be objectively measured:

> In order to measure, things have to be broken down into smaller and smaller units. The result is often long lists of trivial skills as is frequently encountered in BTEC (Business and Technology

Education Council) programmes and NVQ competency assessments. This can lead to a focus on the parts rather than the whole; on the trivial, rather than the significant. It can lead to an approach to education and assessment which resembles a shopping list. When all the items are ticked, the person has passed the course or has learnt something. The role of overall judgment is sidelined.

Smith (1996, 2005)

Another critic, writing about the rise of a competence approach in medical education in the United Kingdom, writes:

... In terms of assessment, the danger is always that we ask questions related to those things that may be more easily measured, instead of asking the more difficult questions.

Talbot (2004: 588)

The NMC's 'Standards' certainly avoids the worst aspects of the competence approach and a series of atomised actions. For example, the competency concerning leadership, management and team working is broad, though possibly difficult to assess: 'All nurses must be self-aware and recognise how their own values, principles and assumptions may affect their practice. They must maintain their own personal and professional development, learning from experience, through supervision, feedback, reflection and evaluation'. (p. 20)

However, some of the tensions that I suggested shot through 19th century nurse education are still in operation today. There are always voices outside and inside nursing that are sceptical about too much education for nurses. The media attention given to apparent nursing failures in care that I discuss in Chapter 6 has provided the springboard for those who claim that the ambitions of nurses' leaders for a highly educated and high status nursing workforce are misguided, only producing a generation of nurses whose cleverness gets in the way of those classic female qualities of common sense, compassion and willingness to dirty their hands in the bodily realm. Against this the arguments made by those who have promoted the recent move to all-graduate entry to nursing, and the NMC's Standards, centre around the increasing technical complexity of (some of) contemporary health care, increased responsibility (sometimes seen as new tasks requiring a new knowledge base such as medicine prescription) and the need for high-level decision-making skills. The document imagines a health service where nurses have influence:

> Nurses must be equipped to lead, delegate, supervise and challenge other nurses and healthcare professionals. They must be able to develop practice, and promote and sustain change. As graduates they must be able to think analytically, use problem-solving approaches and evidence in decision-making, keep up with technical advances and meet future expectations. (p. 4)

Did you know? In 2008–2009 the costs associated with pre-registration training and support were estimated by the Department of Health as almost £1 billion, comprising over £568 million for tuition costs and over £352 million for bursaries.

Prime Minister's Commission (2010)

As a flashback to the effects of Project 2000 in the early 1990s, it should not come as a surprise that many NHS employers are, in the light of degree level registration for nursing, reconsidering their workforce profile as part of a desire to reduce the overall wage bill and in pursuit of the 'flexible' workforce – having workers on hand, who can be hired and trained relatively quickly with exactly the right skills to play a part as each patient moves through the processes of care. I discuss the healthcare division of labour more fully in Chapter 4. The role of nurse as manager and overseer of care is certainly a daily experience for many already, and almost inevitably will grow, yet the NMC's document simultaneously emphasises the nurse as the deliverer of 'high quality essential care to all' (Nursing and Midwifery Council 2010: 5) while suggesting that nursing goes far beyond that. There is another tension here. The rising cost, level of qualification and, possibly, status of nurses will almost inevitably change their role in the overall division of labour in healthcare organisations. They will increasingly supervise care given by others. But the public, politicians and the nursing profession itself all are committed to the idea(l) of the nurse as defined by the delivery of personal care to their patients. So we will see a kind of doubletalk from nursing bodies for a while. They know the reality of trends in healthcare delivery but cannot afford to let go of stereotypical ideas of the caring nurse because it is too valuable a currency to lose. The recent policy documents that I have discussed in this chapter all talk about nurses as delivering 'high quality, compassionate and complex care' to their patients. It is true but it is not the whole story.

UK nurse education has taken the difficult journey from the convent-like discipline of the 19th and early 20th century, through the trade-based training of the middle years of the last century, simultaneously supplying a significant proportion of the workforce, to being taken into an expanding university sector. There has not always been consensus within nursing about the best place and the right emphasis for nurse education. Strident voices outside the profession have suggested that the ambition for high levels of education is part of the problem in nursing rather than the solution. Nursing's leaders have, so far successfully, persuaded the government and some of the public that the complexity of nursing work calls for higher levels of preparation than previously required.[6] Finally, nursing has something to be pleased about. However, this success comes at the cost of possibly reducing numbers of qualified nurses in the workforce and of an increasingly supervisory role for those who are

---

[6] At the time of writing, and prompted by the poor press that the profession is currently receiving, the RCN engaged Lord Willis to manage a consultation on nurse education. It supported degree education but found student support in placements uneven.

there. It is up to you to decide whether this is a price worth paying. What the individual who participates in degree level nurse education gets is, I would argue, definitely worth the price: an almost certainly more in-depth and thorough preparation for practice with opportunities to think critically and be involved in high-quality debate that leaders in health care, confident practitioners and citizens, more generally, need more than ever.

3

Who Regulates Nursing and Why?
The NMC and Its Predecessors

The regulation of health professionals in the United Kingdom is largely one of state-sanctioned self-regulation. Individuals wanting to use titles such as 'registered medical practitioner' or 'midwife' must be registered with the respective professional council, otherwise they can face prosecution. State regulation of the major health professions is taken for granted today but Florence Nightingale, for one, did not envision a nursing that had this kind of state involvement. State regulation is an attractive achievement for professions, offering protection for the title that practitioners use or a monopoly over a particular area of work. The regulation of medicine in the United Kingdom began in the 19th century and has been a successful model emulated by other aspiring professions, including nursing. However, nursing's moves toward regulation have been dogged by division. Recent UK governments, in the context of increasing consumerism and high profile medical and, to a lesser extent, nursing scandals, have increased the state's influence over the regulation of these professions. This chapter discusses the various reviews of nursing and midwifery regulation undertaken by consulting companies, the demise of the UKCC and the experiences of its troubled successor, the Nursing and Midwifery Council (NMC), as well as the creation of the Council for Healthcare Regulatory Excellence (CHRE) in 2002 which 'regulates the regulators'. It discusses what this means for practising nurses. It concludes nurses are responsible but not autonomous.

To work in the United Kingdom, all nurses, midwives and specialist community public health nurses must register with the NMC and renew their registration every 3 years. As a professional, you are in the public eye. Anyone can search 'the register' on the web to check if you are genuine, and anyone can look to see if you are facing discipline by the regulator and what the charge against you is (see Chapter 6 for more about the discipline of poorly performing nurses). The NMC will have largely shaped the course you are required to take to become eligible to register as a nurse, and it sets out what you need to do to stay practising as one. This is professional regulation. It has been considered a great prize for a professional group to achieve this kind of state-sanctioned regulation, but, increasingly, it comes at a price. And at a time when scandalous failures in health care are making the news with puzzling regularity, professional regulation is under uncomfortable scrutiny. Even as I write this paragraph, the NMC's Chief Executive has just announced his resignation, taking the number of heads of that body to 5 in 6 years, and now the regulator has received a blistering review finding it 'failing at every level' (Ford 2012) at the same moment that it is proposing a significant increase in fees.

In this chapter, I set out what professional self-regulation is and how its character has been challenged and changed in recent years, and what this means for the practising nurse. Like many writers on this topic, I use medical regulation in the United Kingdom as a reference point.

Let's agree to call a profession 'a special kind of knowledge-based occupation'.[1] The major professions in most developed countries enter into a pact with their governments. The professions get a licence from the state to practice. In – supposedly – everyone's best interests, the professions are permitted to draw a boundary around their area of work and are granted a monopoly inside this boundary. They grant entry into the field via selection, examination and certification and keep everyone else out. However, or perhaps, in return,

---

[1] This minimal definition as well as much of the opening discussion of professions and professional self-regulation is informed by Judith Allsop and Mike Saks' book *Regulating the Health Professions*. Allsop, J. and M. Saks, Eds. (2002). *Regulating the Health Professions*. London, Sage.

the major professions do the work of the state. Most modern states could not function without an extensive healthcare system or without a legal system. It is the decisions of doctors, for example, that determine eligibility for certain state benefits, or whether a disturbed individual can be detained in a mental hospital against their will. Marxists would say that the professions serve the interests of the structures of capital. The professions are protected to such an extent that it is usually illegal for someone without the training endorsed by the relevant regulator, let's say as a doctor, to claim to be a doctor or do the work of a doctor. This has the benefit of protecting the public from bogus and possibly dangerous impostors (though it doesn't protect the public from possibly dangerous genuine doctors). In most cases this level of market closure enables professions to gain considerable status, income and power. In addition, the pact includes (or has included) the ability for the professions to regulate themselves. In other words, they can set their own standards for behaviour, usually expressed in a code of practice, and punish those within the profession whom they judge to have fallen short. More recently they have introduced requirements that practitioners need to demonstrate continuing competence.

Regulation can be statutory or voluntary. Statutory regulators have legal powers to make registration obligatory, and the disciplinary decisions they take, such as striking a practitioner off its register, are recognised in law. Voluntary regulators do not have legal enforcement powers, but instead encourage professional recognition and responsibility through voluntary registration against agreed standards (NMC_Admin 2011).

The regulatory bodies such as the General Medical Council (GMC) and NMC have to balance the requirements of, and pressure from, three different groups: their own members whose professional fees[2] pay the

---

[2] At the time of writing, nurses have to pay £76 per year registration fee. At less than the price of a nice pair of shoes, it's a bargain. But a rise to over £100 is coming.

bills, the public at large who look to these bodies to maintain standards and protect them against poor practice, punishing perpetrators once malpractice has been proved, and the government who hold, in theory at least, ultimate power over them. This assumption that the regulatory bodies make decisions in the interests of the public as a whole, rather than their membership, differentiates them from professional associations like the RCN or British Medical Association (BMA).

Medicine is seen as one of the highly successful professions and the way it interacts with the state has been taken as a model by other professional groups. In the United Kingdom, the GMC was established in 1858, well before the days of the first Ministry of Health (the Ministry of Health was formed in 1919), let alone a National Health Service (1948). Acting first to establish rather than maintain occupational closure, its chief role was distinguishing those practitioners who had followed an approved course of preparation from those who had not. This simultaneously identified to the public, in theory at least, which practitioners could be trusted while keeping competitors, 'quacks', out of the area. As with many things Victorian, the emphasis within the medical establishment and what became the GMC was on a loosely defined uprightness of character that marked out doctors not only from their clients but from the brute world of industry and commerce.[3] Its way of working has often been described as something like a gentleman's club. Informal judgements about the moral, and inextricably, social qualities of doctors would ensure that they acted always in the best interests of their patients. This was early professional self-regulation.

---

[3] Celia Davies describes the development of professional self-regulation in medicine as 'a project of nineteenth-century middle-class masculinity', built up and reinforcing the fantasy of masculinity as detached and self-reliant, apparently autonomous. Davies, C. (2002). What about the girl next door? Gender and the politics of professional self-regulation. *Gender, Health and Healing: The Public/Private Divide*. G. Bendelow, M. Carpenter, C. Vautier and S. Williams. London, Routledge.

Why registration?

The success of medical regulation, it is generally thought, provided the impetus for nurses in the 19th century to pursue the same goal. Those nurses campaigning for state registration saw better education and training of nurses, uniformity of a nursing curriculum and recognition of approved training schools attached to sufficiently substantial hospitals among their aims (Rafferty 1996).[4] But nursing registration was dogged with conflict between those with different interests and by domineering characters from its early days. Lack of sponsorship at government level and lack of support from the influential voluntary hospitals that feared a loss of control over standards of training and discipline, followed by the interruption of the First World War meant that the General Nursing Council which established the nursing register was not formed until well into the 20th century (1919).[5] In order to achieve any credibility, existing groups of practising nurses needed to be persuaded to join the register. The size of the nursing workforce and the volume of work needed to be done by the council caused backlogs. In the 4 months following the opening of the register, 3,235 applications were received but only 984 were completed. Five months later only 1,550 out of an estimated 50,000 nurses were registered. In 1920 it cost a nurse one guinea (the literal equivalent is £1.05, in average earnings worth approximately £100 today) to join the register and 2s 6d (12½pence) each year to remain there.

After initial tribulations in which most of the council members resigned, the GNC set about establishing the first national syllabus and standards for examination for nurse training.

---

[4] Much of the material for this section comes from Anne Marie Rafferty's book. Rafferty, A. M. (1996). *The Politics of Nursing Knowledge*. London, Routledge.

[5] The NMC website includes a brief account of its history, The History of Nursing and Midwifery Regulation; From 1860 to the present – how we got to where we are today. At the time of writing this can be found at http://www.nmc-uk.org/About-us/The-history-of-nursing-and-midwifery-regulation/ Midwives have been regulated under statutory professional self-regulation since 1902.

Many believed that improving the standard of training for nurses would raise the reputation of the profession, improve recruitment and screen out unsuitable candidates – such as those whose level of literacy meant they could scarcely write a report on their patients. Nevertheless, by now operating within the harsh economic downturn of the 1920s, the GNC was unable to realise its proposed standard national curriculum. As the 1930s wore on, the GNC faced another similar problem to today in terms of perceived difficulty in recruitment to the profession and attrition from training. Hospitals lost half of their trainees each year and had to re-recruit to restore their numbers. As today, most are lost in the first year of training, and many probationers found difficulty in coping with the combination of theoretical training and work on the wards.

So the early days of the GNC saw a series of internal conflicts which individual government ministers and others were repeatedly called to solve, sometimes much to their irritation. Yet from today's perspective, the GNC was a survivor, with a working lifetime of 60 years. But it was a growing sense of troubles in nursing during the 1960s that set in train the process that replaced it with new regulatory arrangements that lasted barely one-third of this time. The 1960s witnessed growing concerns about the status of nurses in the NHS, poor career structures for senior nurses, high levels of turnover, dissatisfaction with the structure and usefulness of the profession's basic training as well as calls for improved pay and conditions. It was in this context of unrest that the Labour government of the day announced the establishment of a committee on nursing under the chairmanship of Asa Briggs, a historian and Vice-Chancellor at the University of Sussex (Davies and Beach 2000). The resulting Briggs Report from 1972 became a major landmark for the profession. Its diagnosis of the profession was in some ways bleak, yet many nurses welcomed the fact that at last the profession was receiving some attention from the government. I discussed its effect on nurse education in the previous chapter.

The report's discussion of professional regulation only featured on 10 of its 220 pages (Davies and Beach 2000), yet it ushered in the way for the body (or bodies) that replaced the GNC. The proposals – for a UK-wide Central Council and an educational board for each of the four countries of the United Kingdom – provoked debate and exposed nursing as, once more, a fractured profession with nurses, midwives and health visitors along with nurse managers, educators and different grades of nurse having different interests. In spite of this the 1979 Nurses, Midwives and Health Visitors Act brought together these professions under a single regulator and onto a single register. The council, appointed by the Secretary of State, was heavily weighed with nurses – 27 of the 33 were nurses, midwives or health visitors. Only six members were drawn from outside the profession. Of these, two were doctors and the so-called lay members were chosen for their educational or financial backgrounds. Its first chief executive was the existing registrar of the GNC for England and Wales. It is clear that the government's assumption, unlike today, was that the profession could and should be self-regulating. The members of each National Board were to be elected every 5 years. The UKCC's task was 'to establish and improve standards' of education and professional conduct. The actual combining of previously separate registers into one was a huge task involving dealing with up to 1.25 million records, many of which related to nurses who had changed their name upon marriage. And for the first time, the regulator could remove a nurse from the register for unfitness to practice on the grounds of ill-health. Other aspects of the UKCC's regulatory powers seem weighed toward the professional from today's perspective, and JM Consulting's review nearly 20 years later noted that the 1997 Act did not make public protection its main explicit aim (JM Consulting Ltd. 1998: 31). The council made it clear that the primary purposes of disciplinary processes were not to be punitive; the body maintained its association with the Nurses' Welfare Service, set up to support nurses undergoing disciplinary procedures, and those making a complaint about a nurse had no right of appeal if the National Boards did not refer the case to the UKCC. When the council formally started its work in 1982, it faced a considerable backlog of professional conduct cases, a problem that has never gone away for the nursing regulator.

Seven years later, the organisation and functioning of the five statutory bodies was reviewed. This led to the 1992 Act and changes in legislation – the UKCC became a directly elected body and the National Boards became smaller, executive bodies appointed by the respective Secretaries of State (and, for Northern Ireland, the Head of the Department of Health and Social Services for Northern Ireland). All professional conduct functions were transferred to the Central Council (JM Consulting Ltd. 1998: 31). The year 1992 also saw the publication of the UKCC's new framework for professional accountability – the Scope of Professional Practice. It placed the onus on the individual nurse to work within the limits of their personal knowledge and ability as well as to do something about any deficits. It also warned nurses and midwives against inappropriate delegation to others that would not be in the best interests of patients and clients.

Medical and nursing regulation in the late 20th century

Statutory professional self-regulation must be able to justify itself compared with other types of regulation. The emphasis on public protection must be, and be perceived to be, its prime purpose. The current perception by many professionals and the public is that this type of regulation places emphasis on protecting the professions. Whilst the current statutory bodies themselves are conscious of their primary public protection role, others are not.

JM Consulting Ltd. (1998: 40)

Returning to medical regulation, some have said that its 19th century principles, because they were so entrenched in the British establishment, endured for a century or more. It was not until the 1980s that a UK government even began to examine the performance of doctors in the health service, let alone interfere in medical discipline. The Conservative government of Margaret Thatcher, which was in some ways no respecter of tradition, gave the structure and workings of the NHS considerable attention (see Chapter 7) but did not directly tackle professional self-regulation. However, toward the end of its time in office it commissioned management consultants

JM Consulting to look at possible changes to the way that what are now generally referred to as the allied health professions (AHPs), plus some others, were regulated. Medical regulation was not challenged. In 1997, 3 months into their government, New Labour used the same consultants to carry out a review of the regulation of nursing (JM Consulting Ltd. 1998).[6] The resulting report's main criticism was that nursing and midwifery regulation was too inward looking and that its workings had inadequate lay involvement. They saw this degree of insularity as outmoded in a society where it was no longer reasonable to consider that the public had inadequate knowledge of the work of professionals to participate in their regulation on a par with them. The report's repeated assertion was that the primary duty of professional regulators is to protect the public.

The review recommended that nursing registration be dependent on a statement of good character, satisfactory criminal record checks, evidence of continuing professional development and written acceptance of a code of conduct (p. 284). It also recommended fewer council members, one-third of whom should be from outside the profession and selected by a government appointments commission. The new council was warned not to be 'overly sympathetic' to professionals but to work in partnership with employers, and some have noted that senior NHS managers were heavily represented on the new council (Cooke 2012). One of the themes running through this book is the tension between the state and powerful professional groups. From the viewpoint of that conflict, certain important contextual events made erosions into professional self-regulation more achievable for governments. The late 1990s marked a period of exposures of medical misconduct and scandals and the apparently inadequate way that this was handled by the GMC. The Bristol Royal Infirmary scandal was in the headlines and the crimes of GP Harold Shipman, who murdered an undetermined number of his patients (probably over 200), were emerging. There was pressure,

---

[6] At the time of writing, this report is available from the English Department of Health website at http://www.dh.gov.uk/en/Publicationsandstatistics/Publications/PublicationsLegislation/DH_4006034.

for example in a leader in the *Times* newspaper, for the independent inspection of doctors (17th November 1998). As mentioned
in Chapter 1, trust in traditional authority figures had been wearing
thin in many Western countries, and many governments looked to
the transparency of procedures and processes to replace that lost
trust (see Chapter 5 on the rise of evidence-based health care).
Increased involvement in the regulation of the professions was managed at a time when it was likely to receive a high degree of popular
support.

Some have seen the state and NHS managers in an alliance
which has encroached on the autonomy of the health professions
to enhance its own ability to direct health services. The UKCC
had on occasion made itself unpopular with managers by raising
concerns about the environment of care, particularly in relation to
the nursing home sector. Senior managers interviewed by Hannah
Cooke in the late 1990s and early 2000s were highly critical of the
UKCC, on occasion describing the members of its various panels
as 'idiots'. Managers, she says, felt that if they had sacked a member of staff the UKCC should back their decision rather than ask
what most people would assume to be important questions about
the context such as training availability and workload issues (Cooke
2006, 2012). Interestingly, JM Consulting recommended that the
new Council (the NMC) should provide systematic feedback to
employers about 'lessons that can be learnt from cases, and particularly where features of the working environment were contributing
to misconduct or poor performance' (p. 22). In practice, there is an
artificial separation between the remit of professional regulators like
the NMC with their focus on individual wrongdoing and the work
originally of the Commission for Healthcare Improvement founded
in 2001 (closed in 2004 and its work transferred to the Healthcare
Commission, now, in turn the Care Quality Commission[7]), which

---

[7] It seems that regulation of health care in the United Kingdom is characterised by
constant review, critique from governments, dissatisfaction from the public and the
media and a constant turnover of organisations and their chief executives.

is charged to 'regulate' system-type failures in healthcare organisations. Most health care, however, emerges from a kind of middle ground of collective activity, shaped partly by organisational procedures, and partly by the individual responsibility of practitioners but, in a complex but crucial way, by the culture and style of the groups involved.

JM Consulting was also concerned about support workers. They represented a vast workforce, estimated at around 800,000 in 1998, but they received a varied training, often worked part-time or in a temporary capacity, often changed job and, of course, were unregulated. Formally support workers were supervised by registered practitioners. The report also noted with alarm that it was known for nurses who had been struck off the register to start work 'immediately' as support workers. There has been continuing controversy over whether such 'non-professional' workers should be subject to some degree of regulation, and if so, by whom. The report recommended that the United Kingdom's health departments 'develop arrangements to regulate healthcare workers' and the debate continues. The recently resigned Chief Executive of the NMC was seen as a strong advocate for support worker regulation – perhaps too strong for some.

As a result of their recommendations, in 2002 the new NMC took over the work of the UKCC. The NMC also inherited its not inconsiderable financial debts (Table 3.1).

Since its inauguration the NMC has experienced a certain amount of turbulence, and today its future hangs in the balance. It has been reviewed, sometimes highly critically, a number of times, resulting in a series of resignations of its chief executives and other key officials. If this were not bad enough, allegations of bullying and racism and dysfunctionality within the organisation were also made in Parliament (Staines 2008).[8]

---

[8] A transcription of the spirited debate about these problems between MP Jim Devine and others at Westminster Hall (16th July 2008) is available at: http://www. theyworkforyou.com/whall/?id=2008-07-16b.120.0 In it we hear the familiar situation of the disciplining by an organisation of individuals who see themselves as whistle-blowers, 'the good guys' as Jim Devine describes them.

Table 3.1 History of regulation in nursing and midwifery in the United Kingdom

Year	Act of Parliament	Comments
1902	Midwives Act	Registration of midwives
1919		Earliest nurse registration by GNC
1962	Health Visiting and Social Work Training Act	Prior to this act, health visiting was restricted to qualified nurses
1979	Nurses, Midwives and Health Visitors Act	Brought professions together under UKCC: 'An Act to establish a Central Council for Nursing, Midwifery and Health Visiting, and National Boards for the four parts of the United Kingdom; to make new provision with respect to the education, training, regulation and discipline of nurses, midwives and health visitors and the maintenance of a single professional register;' implemented in 1983
1992	(Another) Nurses, Midwives and Health Visitors Act (repealed in 1997)	National Boards assume executive responsibility for education and cease to undertake preliminary investigations of misconduct, a role assumed in full by UKCC
1997	(Yet another) Nurses, Midwives and Health Visitors Act	Consolidated the Nurses, Midwives and Health Visitors Act 1979
2001	The Nursing and Midwifery Order	Established the NMC

Based on and expanded from Tremblay (1998: 3) and from www.legislation.gov.uk website which lists and contains texts of the UK legislation.

In 2008 CHRE published a review of the Council's work.[9] It identified a number of problems with the training and appraisal of its committee members, its fitness to practice processes, record keeping of decision-making and speed of processing case work, among others. The report made uncomfortable reading. Shortly afterwards its Chief Executive, Sarah Thewlis, and President, Nancy Kirkland, announced their intention to resign. Nancy Kirkland had only been in post for 8 months. In 2009 the NMC launched a new, reconstituted Council with seven lay and seven professional members.[10] This was the NMC's first fully appointed Council. The Council's term of office began on 1 January 2009, and the Council held its first meeting on 15 January 2009. In 2010 CHRE published an audit which was critical of the NMC's fitness to practise systems. The NMC responded saying that the audit only examined data which was a year out of date and did not acknowledge improvements made since that time.[11] In 2011 CHRE reported again on progress at the Council (CHRE 2011). There had been some change but also problems and lack of stability. Their report noted that during the previous 2 years, the NMC had had three chief executives and three directors of fitness to practise. In a predictable pattern this report in turn was followed by the resignation of Dickon Weir-Hughes, the Council's Chief Executive. His resignation was followed in a matter of months by the resignation of the Council's Chair, Tony Hazell. The Council has just gone through a further review, with the CHRE scrutinising its 'internal structures' and in another highly critical report, the NMC was advised to stick to its core fitness to practice functions and not be distracted by issues such as the regulation of healthcare support workers. There is also the possibility that nurses, doctors

---

[9] The CHRE produced a number of reports on the NMC: *Special Report to the Minister of State for Health Services on the Nursing and Midwifery Council* published in June 2008 and *Fitness to Practise Audit Report* published in February 2010.

[10] The proportion of professionals to lay members finally got to 50/50.

[11] This response, along with an archive of press releases from the NMC can be found on the NMC website, currently at http://www.nmc-uk.org/Press-and-media/News-archive/?p=0.

Table 3.2 Chief executives of the Nursing and Midwifery Council

2012–2013	(Interim Chief Executive) Jackie Smith
2009–2012	Dickon Weir-Hughes
2009	Kathy George from 1 March 2009
2008–2009	Interim Chief Executive, Graham Smith from September 2008
2002–2008	Sarah Thewlis

and other healthcare professionals will all be regulated under a single legislative framework at some point in the future (Sprinks 2012). However, at the time of writing, the future looks uncertain for this troubled body (Table 3.2).

It is hard to know how the NMC and the government will break out of this destructive cycle unless the Council gives up any pretence of independent professional self-regulation. The numbers of nurses among its senior officers seems to be diminishing, and the new Chair appointed by the government in July 2012 was a former senior civil servant with a reputation for rescuing failing organisations. It is hard to see that the NMC's problems, as far as the government are concerned, are simply about administrative inefficiency and not without any connection to some incompatibility of agendas between the government and different factions within nursing.

Some believe that what we are moving to, or have moved to already, is state regulation of nursing and midwifery, rather than self-regulation. If this is true, one potential problem is that a conflict of interest arises between the state both as regulator and as employer (of nurses). In theory, at least, undue state influence over the operation and processes of the regulator could influence outcomes in a way that is more agreeable to the state. As I suggest in Chapter 6, it is sometimes clearly politically expedient to blame nursing or another profession rather than accept the existence of structural failings in the healthcare system, perhaps even failings in part brought about by state action. It is hard to know how far the NMC is bringing about its own demise though continued internal disputes or whether its operation and leadership have been made almost impossible by external forces.

What professional regulation means for the nurse (or student nurse)

So, the bodies that regulate nursing have, since their first days, been dogged by problems, huge administrative challenges, internal divisions and pressure from governments. Sometimes they have not set the best example for the profession in terms of properly handling the tension between responding to individual concerns among its senior staff and dealing with organisational constraints and weaknesses. Nevertheless, the Council, as all regulators do, publishes a code of conduct, and the current nursing and midwifery code was launched in 2008. Probably central to the whole code is the notion of personal responsibility, for example: 'As a professional, you are personally accountable for actions and omissions in your practice and must always be able to justify your decisions' (NMC 2008). It expands: 'If a nurse or midwife is asked to deliver care they consider unsafe or harmful to a person in their care, they should carefully consider their actions and raise their concerns to the appropriate person. Nurses and midwives must act in the best interest of the person in their care at all times'. This is the classic professional doctrine. But at the same time as being true – that is that healthcare professionals have to be considered personally accountable – the complexity of much healthcare delivery can constrain, compromise, distort and distance any actual decision making and conduct by actors in the healthcare arena. Individual nurses are not always powerful actors in healthcare settings and are possibly easy prey to those more powerful individuals (those with positional power or those practised in manipulative techniques i.e. bullies), or powerful cultures, which have come to act in ways that benefit themselves over and above patients or clients. In Chapter 6 I show examples of nurses' acquiescence to poor care. The other manifestation of this lack of power can be found in the actions of those nurses who might avoid accepting responsibility for decision making. So the opposing dangers for nursing are the refusal to accept responsibility or acknowledge decision-making agency on the one hand, and belief in an exaggerated sense of 'autonomy' that fails to appreciate the interdependence and context of all human, and certainly healthcare delivery, actions on the other. Perhaps the best summary is that as a working nurse you are responsible – but not autonomous.

If other professionals involved in health care, doctors, managers and other nurses all practice in line with their own codes, then it should be relatively easy for the individual nurse to practice within the NMC's code. But as soon as anyone's actions drift outside, particularly if this is endorsed by a hierarchy within an organisation, then a difficult tension is introduced for the practising nurse. Then you face the choice: to whistle-blow, to acquiesce – or to move away.

Summary

Professional self regulation is the bargain between the professions and the state. The work of the state is done by well-trained and well-trusted groups. In return the professions police themselves and gain the sometimes considerable benefits of state endorsed monopoly. But the interests of the professions and the state have been prized apart in recent decades. With a sleight of hand, governments have managed to draw more powers back to themselves while claiming to be doing precisely the opposite – devolving powers to the local and specialist groups that have the intimate knowledge of client need. But the health professions, despite presenting themselves as acting in their individual patients' interests, at a structural level should not be trusted alone to organise the configuration of healthcare delivery as they will inevitably attempt to gain more and more power and control. Today we are in a situation where the professions are one of a number of countervailing powers, potentially dominating groups held in tension with the activities of others: the state, employers, patient groups and other professions (Light 1995). This shift and this tension have been at work in the regulation of nursing and midwifery since the days of its first Council in the early 20th century. Today nursing regulation is at another uncomfortable juncture; perhaps about to lose some of the control over its professional destiny it has gained. However, at a time of increasing work pressure on individual nurses within an increasingly pressurised NHS, there has never been a more urgent need for a regulator that can stand against both professional dominance and state control.

4

Nursing's Neighbours: Doctors and Healthcare Support Workers

Nurses work alongside many other healthcare employees, each with a range of special skills. But there is also a hierarchy in healthcare work in terms of power, prestige and reward. It is possible to see nursing placed between medicine and support workers in this hierarchy. Medicine is sometimes the elephant in the room when nurses publicly discuss their practice, as medicine sets the framework for much nursing work and some nurses are ambivalent about acknowledging this. Likewise, much work that was once done by nurses is now carried out by so-called non-professional workers – healthcare support workers (HCSWs) and assistant practitioners (APs) – and managed by nurses. Carers who are unpaid and patients themselves are also expected to work. This chapter discusses the changing relationship between nursing and medicine at a policy, professional and everyday level and between nurses and support workers. The chapter also discusses the way that certain work has, over time, shifted across the boundaries between medicine and nursing and nursing and support workers and argues that this has often been driven by factors external to the work of those occupational groups. It could be hazardous to try to define an essence of nursing because of its shifting character, both across time and between settings. The chapter provides readers with a realistic understanding of the work of both of these groups of neighbouring workers. A discussion of 'teamwork' and its promotion by policy makers is also provided.

How can we think about healthcare work and the people that provide it? One way is to imagine health care as delivered by a team of people, each with their own special area of knowledge and skill and a sphere of work matched to that knowledge and skill. So a speech and language therapist, for example, is the member of this team who works with a patient after a stroke to learn to swallow and speak again; a doctor is the person who makes an initial diagnosis that puts a patient in a particular category and determines the path they take through the healthcare system; a nurse manages the treatment of a patient, monitoring their condition, administering medicines or other treatments and perhaps organising whole services; support workers attend to the detail of patient monitoring and treatment and carry out physical care of patients; administrators organise scheduling, manage records and patient appointments; managers attend to workforce and workflow issues and perhaps make strategic decisions about the whole configuration of a healthcare organisation. Plenty has been written about teams and teamwork, often along the lines of teams working best when members' roles are clear to everyone, when the team has shared objectives and each member values the unique contribution of the others, sometimes in an 'equal but different' approach. Sometimes writers talk about every team member giving up a little bit of autonomy to make the team function properly, and sometimes they say that every team needs a leader. Teamwork is a priority in contemporary talk about healthcare delivery.[1]

But there are other ways to imagine health care. One is to see the healthcare professions spread out in a hierarchy from those with the most power over decision making and the most prestige to those with a very limited sphere of control and the least prestige. Adopting

---

[1] For a summary of features of apparently effective teams, see Mickan, S. and S. Rodger (2005). 'Effective Health Care Teams: A Model of Six Characteristics Developed From Shared Perceptions.' *Journal of Interprofessional Care* **19**(4): 358–370. For a more critical piece of research, see Finn, R., M. Learmonth, et al. (2010). 'Some Unintended Effects of Teamwork in Healthcare.' *Social Science & Medicine* **70**(8): 1148–1154. Finn and colleagues suggest that the teamworking imperative can actually intensify the very professional divisions it sets out to bridge as workers look for ways to preserve the sense of professional identity that they might see teamworking as challenging. The RCN has produced a guide for nurses involved in teams NHS Institute for Innovation and Improvement and Royal College of Nursing (2007). *Developing and Sustaining Effective Teams*. London, RCN.

this view, one might have medical consultants at the top. Not only do they determine the course of treatment for individual patients but medicine is uniquely authorised to determine who is ill and who is not, and the very categories of disease used by most health workers and the public have been largely developed by medicine. Continuing, all the other workers would be 'paramedical' or 'allied to medicine', carrying out the work determined by doctors, supporting medical work. Until perhaps the mid-1980s 'administrators', by which I mean the people now largely known as managers, would also be seen as supporting the work of medicine. However, more recently they might be understood as responsible for the overall machinery and conduct of health care (see next approach). Writers investigating health care from this point of view have studied how professions gain and attempt to maintain power, how the boundaries between them are managed and what determines whether a new occupational group can gain the much-prized status of profession. I covered some of this ground in Chapter 3 when discussing professional regulation and have more to say in this chapter.

A third approach to understanding healthcare work is a variant of the first in that it concerns matching different aspects of the work to workers with different skills. However the emphasis is not on the broadly autonomous team of different professionals but is more managerially driven. In the previous two approaches, the existing professional groups are taken as given and as the starting point for healthcare work – for example there is 'medical' work or 'nursing' work. With this managerial approach, it is the need of the organisation to deal with its patients in the most efficient and effective way that comes first. (What is best for the organisation may or may not be the same as what its patients want.) A manager taking a fresh look at this might think that the existing divisions of work into that done by the various (sometimes expensive) professional groups actually hinders the best delivery of health care, and that what is needed is fewer groups who can do more things. (Government documents, for example the NHS Plan, have seen 'traditional hierarchical ways of working' as a major hindrance to efficiency and innovation in the NHS.) The manager would, in their ideal world, hire exactly the workers needed to get the work done and have influence over the training and skills that each comes with. The rise of APs in recent years is evidence of this approach. In a health service currently facing enormous financial pressures, we are seeing much more attention to this approach.

Consider these UK workforce statistics: It takes 5–6 years to train a doctor, and basic training costs approximately £274,000. Nurses take 3 years to train at an approximate total cost of £45,224.[2] Assistant practitioners usually undertake a 2-year 'Foundation Degree' on a day a week basis. Healthcare support workers get hugely variable training ranging from a matter of weeks to over a year.

I am going to start by elaborating the second model – of professional dominance and struggles for power – because, out of my three, it is the way of understanding professional work with the longest tradition and will give us a better perspective on the other two. The simplest daily interaction of individual professionals and the most apparently casual organisational arrangements and national structural planning such as who is included and who is not included in Agenda for Change[3] can only be fully understood with some knowledge of this field of thinking.

Professional status and power in nursing and medicine

In the last chapter I talked about what a profession is, about how the major professions, like medicine, successfully gain exclusive right to work in a certain area and exclude rivals. Those who have studied the character of professional work have devoted far more attention to medicine than to nursing.[4] When nursing has been examined, it has

---

[2] These figures are based on Curtis, L. (2010). *Unit Costs of Health and Social Care 2010*. Canterbury, Personal Social Services Research Unit.

[3] Doctors, dentists and senior managers are not included in Agenda for Change.

[4] If you are interested in one possible explanation, see Strong, P. (1984). 'Viewpoint: The Academic Encirclement of Medicine?' *Sociology of Health & Illness* **6**(3): 339–358. He argues that medical sociologists hoped that some of the prestige of doctors might rub off.

tended to be compared to one of the most established professions and has been labelled a 'semi-profession' (Etzioni 1969). Because nurses and doctors work in the same area, it is almost unavoidable to compare medicine and nursing in terms of their professional status. This sense of differential status, and sometimes a sense of injustice about this, has fuelled a drive to raise the status of nursing from its early days.

In response to the fear that too much emphasis on character risks devaluing the professional and technical competence of nurses, a number of nurse leaders, particularly in the United States, set out the call for the development of a formalised nursing knowledge base, as one said, 'speedily defined and organised as nursing science' (Bixler and Bixler 1945: 730). The 1950s, 1960s and 1970s saw an enthusiastic answer to this call. A number of systems of 'nursing' knowledge emerged, many prefaced explicitly as providing a credential for professional status. The aim of such an enterprise, according to those leading it, was the desire to develop a range of 'concepts' that were distinct from those in use within medicine and to differentiate them from those of other disciplines (Meleis 1985).

From today's perspective, the belief that the identification of a unique field of knowledge for the profession would be followed by an increase in status and recognition seems naïve. Back in the 1960s, Fred Katz argued that nursing leaders failed to understand that professional status depends not only on the possession of a body of knowledge but also requires that other groups, social and professional, acknowledge the legitimacy of that knowledge. Writing in Etzioni's much-quoted collection of essays on the 'semi-professions' (Etzioni 1969) (which included discussions of social work and teaching), he claimed that a rigid caste system in hospitals separated nurses from doctors and resulted in nurses carrying out doctor's orders. In his view, a 'drastic rearrangement of social roles in the hospital' would have to occur before physicians and hospital administrators would be prepared to acknowledge this (Katz 1969). Katz's analysis is old and draws its conclusions sometimes on limited, unpublished and already dated empirical research. He concluded that the nurse 'has no clearly formulated body of professional knowledge that is recognized and accepted by others' (p. 62).

What do you know? Katz's statement was written about 45 years ago and clearly much has changed since then in society and in health care, but, if you disagree with Katz's diagnosis, it is worth asking what exactly this body of professional knowledge is made up of.

Many studies of medicine focus on the idea of medical dominance, arguing that ultimately all the healthcare work that is done by other occupations concerning the patient is organised or authorised by doctors (Freidson 1970). Not only this, but some argue that medicine has so dominated the field that it has significant control over the training of other occupational groups or even influence over whether another occupational group is allowed to develop as a profession at all[5] (Freidson 1994).

Walby and Greenwell (1994) also researched professional differences between doctors and nurses. They did their work during the early 1990s in a UK health service that had recently undergone reforms designed to increase responsiveness to patients while offering increased organisational autonomy in the form of 'independent' trust status (Department of Health 1989). They proposed that nurses were only able to exercise partial autonomy because the scope of their work with patients was set by the initial admission, diagnosis, treatment plan and discharge which was determined by medical consultants. In response to this limitation, they argued, nurses tried to separate out an area of practice where they could exercise more control and described this as 'caring work'. However, as Walby and Greenwell point out, a claim that a separation can be made between the technical 'curing' work of doctors and the 'caring' work of nurses, with its suggestion that doctors are not concerned with caring, is not one that stands up to scrutiny (p. 53). Nevertheless, nursing has continued to strongly identify with 'caring' as its distinctive feature.

---

[5] For example, in the early 20th century some of the first chiropractors were jailed in the United States for 'practicing medicine without a license'.

> **Try this exercise:** When you are next in a healthcare setting, make a note of three interactions between a health professional and a patient that you consider 'caring' (for example someone taking the time to listen, explaining something carefully) and three that appear 'uncaring' (where you think there is a little brusqueness, impatience, working in a way that's convenient for the professional but difficult for a patient). Is there any association between the type of professional and the 'caring' or 'uncaring' interactions?

Some studies of medicine, nursing and professionalism show us the part that gender plays in this arena. One important contribution to this topic is the suggestion that medical ideology promotes a view of professional autonomy that relies on a perhaps characteristic male blindness to the work of, usually female, clerical, nursing and other health service staff that enable doctors to do their job and to have that brief encounter with the patient for which the patient may wait hours or even years (Davies 1995). We could say that the whole notion of being a professional and even working in an organisation at all is 'gendered' male, because it relies on an assumption that the fully committed worker has someone else to service their personal needs (picking up the children from school), and that its bureaucratic features require a kind of impartial, formalised, disembodied, rational ('we must make the best decision for the organisation even if it is painful') approach that many see as reflecting stereotypical male values. Faced with this, it could be that nursing needs a radically different concept of what it is to be a profession.

But what do we know about how nurses and doctors actually interact? The NMC and Department of Health both emphasise the need for nurses to have the qualifications and the confidence to work as equals with other professions in high-level decision-making teams (Department of Health and CNO's Office 2006; Nursing and Midwifery Council 2010). But given the formal hierarchical differences described, the question that many writers who have studied these interactions address is what tactics do nurses actually adopt to influence decisions made by doctors? One early answer was by means of the 'doctor/nurse game' by which a more knowledgeable nurse could indirectly suggest a course of action to an inexperienced junior doctor while preserving the fiction that the doctor is the one deciding (Stein 1967). Other writers have looked at local strategies used by nurses to gain or maintain professional power in the face of medical dominance. These have included the discovery of nurses' use of organisational 'guerrilla' tactics to create a space for control over their work (Salhani and Coulter 2009) and the employment of subversive actions, such as humour or withholding information, to challenge the dominating authority of doctors (Griffiths 1998; Simpson 2007). In the psychiatric ward studied by Salhani, the nursing team ran a parallel therapeutic service that went counter to the official drug-centred approach of the consultant team.

In 2000 the English Chief Nursing Officer (CNO) wrote about new roles for nurses that had been promoted in the NHS Plan. Many of these were previously undertaken by doctors.
   The CNO's 10 key roles for nurses are:

- To order diagnostic investigations
- To make and receive referrals direct
- To admit and discharge patients for specified conditions and within agreed protocols
- To manage patient caseloads
- To run clinics
- To prescribe medicines and treatments
- To carry out a wide range of resuscitation procedures
- To perform minor surgery and outpatient procedures
- To triage patients using the latest IT to the most appropriate health professional
- To take a lead in the way local health services are organised and in the way that they are run.

To sum up, medical power has been studied extensively and nursing rather less. Nursing's leaders have been concerned with the profession's status since its early days. Though many have been aware of a link between knowledge and professional prestige, the profession has an ambivalent approach to formalised 'scientific' knowledge. On the one hand it has been essential, at least since the early decades of the 20th century when nursing was fully accepted into a bureaucratic healthcare system in the United Kingdom, to claim that its activities were based on a sound technical–rational basis. On the other, formalising this basis for knowledge has risked too close an identification with medicine, a comparison in which nursing may well be viewed unfavourably because the extent of its scientific basis may be seen as less extensive. However, too strong an identification with the 'unique caring nature' of nursing work could trap nursing in a role that is not highly valued or rewarded by society. Others have adopted the 'equal but different' approach and emphasised nursing's control over a circumscribed range of work.

Before talking about how healthcare work is constantly moved 'down' this occupational hierarchy, to cheaper workers (or to patients and carers themselves), I talk about the group of workers placed to the other side of nurses in this supposed hierarchy who are receiving considerable attention in today's NHS, healthcare support workers and assistant practitioners.

Healthcare support workers[6]

Unqualified support workers have nearly always worked alongside qualified nurses. In the past student and auxiliary nurses have carried out a great deal of the direct patient work (Allen 2001), but today much of that work is carried out by a growing number of healthcare support workers. The health service has relied on these workers partly for demographic reasons, when it has been difficult to recruit enough nurses, but more obviously because these workers are not only cheaper to employ, but also quicker and cheaper to train. They are on the landscape and they are here to stay. However they have presented a dilemma for nursing. On the one hand professional voices in nursing have emphasised a need to 'reclaim' the direct

---

[6] For much of this section I draw on Davina Allen's insightful examination of the changing shape of nursing work.

hands-on care of patients as a core part of nursing work. And today they are joined by voices outside the profession who criticise nurses for what they see as refusal to attend to this traditional nursing role in preference for more technical or managerial work. On the other hand an increasing managerialist influence in the NHS is moving nurses away from this basic work into more supervisory roles and rebalancing the workforce toward non-professional workers. The immediate drive for this change today appears to be financial, though plenty of NHS managers and politicians insist on denying this. I would suggest that the current financial turbulence provides an opportunity for NHS managers to move toward the vision of the flexible workforce over which they have more control than I outlined in my third model earlier in this chapter.[7]

Earlier I mentioned how professional dominance can extend to one professional group having influence over entry to and the practice of another. The example I gave was of medicine and various 'paramedical' occupations. But it is clear that nursing has or is looking for a similar control regarding healthcare support workers.

---

[7] The development of assistant practitioners can be seen as part of the managerialist drive for a more flexible workforce than the traditional professions provide:

> The NHS Career Framework, reinforced through the NHS pay system, Agenda for Change, introduced a nine-tier framework for career progression within the NHS. This set out a formal progression route that would allow people to enter at any point within the framework (depending on their level of qualification and/or experience) and then to progress and expand their role with further experience and training. The purpose of the career framework was to enable skills escalation and aid the development of new roles to meet patient need. Its other aims were to assist with the development of competence-based workforce planning, give opportunities for individual career planning, enable easier recruitment and retention and improve transferability of roles and skills across healthcare organisations regardless of location. The career framework, therefore, is viewed as supporting earlier developments in workforce redesign introduced to facilitate the design and delivery of care arrangements that would help ameliorate pressures for efficient service delivery whilst meeting patient expectations and preferences.

Skills for Health (2010). *The Role of Assistant Practitioners in the NHS: Factors Affecting Evolution and Development of the Role. Skills for Health Expert Paper.* Bristol, SfH.

The Royal College of Nursing's approach to accepting these workers into its membership gives a sense of a gradual realisation that this growing group need to be wooed in case another organisation gets there first.

> In 2001 the RCN opened the membership to allow healthcare assistants (HCAs) with NQV level three to join.
>
> The RCN expanded its membership criteria to encompass all HCAs reviewing the criteria for membership in 2005. New joining criteria were agreed to include a clearer definition of HCSWs to include all healthcare support workers who: (1) provide health and social care and whose routine work is delegated to them by a registered nurse or midwife or (2) have a qualification in health and care level one of the National Qualifications Framework in England or level three of the Scottish Credit and Qualifications Framework in Scotland.
>
> The membership category for HCAs at these stages was 'Associate', and although HCAs were eligible to vote in a general ballot, branch or forum elections, Council elections and presidential elections they had no representation on the RCN's Council.
>
> At the AGM in October 2011 the vote was passed to enable HCA and assistant practitioner members to become 'full' members, and nominations are sought for two seats on RCN Council, to take up their roles after the AGM in October 2012. Later in 2012 nominations open for places on a governance committee, as the current HCA and AP committee has no governance role at present.
>
> For further details see: http://www.rcn.org.uk/hca.[8]

HCSWs have caused much head scratching among those involved in healthcare policy. Their main concern is that this growing group of workers is diverse in job titles, level of training and in what they actually do. Added to this, unlike nurses and doctors, they are 'unregulated'. For many, including managers who want to solve local patient-flow problems, this diversity might not be a problem, and clearly, by and large, the workers themselves are highly committed

---

[8] I am grateful to Tanis Hand, RCN Health Care Assistant Adviser for this chronology. The interpretation is mine.

and skilled individuals. A useful review of what has been written about these workers (NHS Education for Scotland 2010) identified these themes (Table 4.1):

Table 4.1 The topics and themes identified from the literature

Definitions of HCSWs	Tasks conducted by HCSWs
Evolution of the HCSW role	Job descriptions
Number of HCSWs	Regulation
Characteristics of HCSWs	The impact of HCSWs
Education and training provided for HCSW development	Views of HCSWs on education and the role
Supervision of HCSWs	Views of managers on the role
Mentorship of HCSWs in training	Views of registered practitioners on the role
Relationships with other healthcare workers	Service users' views on the role
Boundary disputes and professional identity	Development into registered roles
Roles and scopes of practice	Future developments
	The assistant practitioner role

Although the review identified a large number of job titles held by this kind of worker, all make it plain they work to someone else's instructions: they are assistants, supporters or associates. The roles have developed in response to local, national or sometimes international drivers. Their numbers are growing: in England in 2008 there were 284,000 full time equivalent (FTE), a significant rise from the equivalent figure of 220,000 (FTE) in 1998. (p. 13)

They tend to be slightly older than registered nurses, more likely to work part time, and more likely to have connections with the local community where they work. Their typical qualification is a National Vocational Qualification (NVQ), though Foundation degrees[9] are

---

[9] The Open University defines these degrees as a short, work-related degree that prepares individuals for a specific type of work.

commonly used to prepare certain support workers for assistant practitioner roles. However, the review noted three problems with vocational training programmes for HCAs. 'Firstly no consistency in their duration, secondly questions over who is responsible for and pays for the training and finally a lack of consensus on the content of the training... [there is] no consensus on the best way of providing minimum standards of training to HCAs' (p. 19). Nevertheless, where educational courses for HCAs have been implemented, they have 'helped achieve an increase in knowledge, confidence and skills' (p. 23).[10]

The report characterised three ways that support workers were deployed: *use*, where most of their work involved direct patient care while registered nurses tended to become more involved in paperwork and discharge planning; *misuse*, where sometimes due to workload pressures they were required to undertake tasks for which they had received no training; or *non-use*, where registered nurses appeared to prevent them from properly putting their skills and experience into practice. Echoing some of the literature mentioned earlier, research has suggested that some registered nurses feel their core role and identity encroached upon by support workers and try to differentiate themselves from them in a number of ways including by emphasising their 'professional qualifications and accountability as registered healthcare professionals; their level of knowledge; their emphasis on patient-centred, holistic care in comparison to their perceptions of HCAs undertaking a task-oriented approach. There is evidence of nurses sensing a loss of relationships with patients and attempting to protect their identity by restricting the roles of HCAs. Equally HCAs may choose to withhold patient and other information from nurses in an attempt to increase their influence' (p. 29). Part of the trouble is that there is confusion, from a certain perspective, over what is 'nursing' work – work 'which should

---

[10] The Department of Health commissioned Skills for Health and Skills for Care to start work in April 2012 on developing national minimum training standards and a code of conduct for healthcare support workers in England.

only be performed by nurses' (p. 31) and what is not. I say more about work at the boundary of professional realms later.

I end this section on support workers by talking about some findings of focus groups I conducted with two groups of HCSWs undertaking courses at my university. The groups were made of those completing an AP course and those undertaking shorter training for HCSWs but not leading to the AP qualification. All were highly motivated and hand-picked by their managers to complete these courses. They were confident about their role and its future. For some the extra qualification would make an immediate change to their salary. Some interesting paradoxes emerged. For example, on the one hand, when asked their view on the current widespread opinion that nurses were becoming too detached from direct patient care, their agreement was overwhelming:

> *Anita*: I agree, I don't think there's enough hands-on care for a lot of nurses now. I think where I work, a lot of nurses take on the junior doctors' roles, to do more. They're just, you know, it's more about you know, they have to make sure the medication's all sorted and everything and you know, leaving all the actual main work to the care workers.
>
> *Vera*: Well no, just like, you know, new nurses coming in will just, you know, not the actual wanting to do the hands-on care.
>
> *Fred*: It's more of an academic qualification now than it is . . . . what's the word, vocation? It's all about the academic side of it, the writing, the essays.
>
> *Anita*: It's too academic

Yet most of the group saw their course as a stepping stone into nurse training, though some were clear that they did not. Plainly something about becoming a nurse was attractive despite the obvious conclusion that if they followed this career, they too would end up with a job dominated by paperwork. The answer for some seemed to do with the respect that a professional qualification might give them, and some spoke of what they felt was disrespectful treatment by some nurses.

A further surprise emerged when the group talked about how they imagined the extra qualification would change their actual day-to-day work. Many felt that their extra qualification would make no difference to their range of work but would provide them background knowledge, an example given was anatomy and physiology, for what they do already. However, this new knowledge would give them a new level of responsibility:

> *Pam*: Because you've got knowledge to back up your practical skills that you can be more autonomous because you'll be able to not just do the task like I said before, you'll understand what you're doing it for, why you're doing it and what impact it can have so that you'll be able to take more responsibility for your actions whereas if you're just doing something, somebody's got to take responsibility for what may happen from you doing that.

However some looked forward to a different role:

> *Rosie*: ... so like [I'll be] getting more jobs and responsibilities, it's really good.
> *Vera*: Being more autonomous, being able to, they're going to set up a clinic for me, to do an assessment clinic, now I'm a band 4 because I've got the knowledge and I understand the conditions and the effects they have on different things; I suppose taking some work away from somebody else to lighten their load but you're now deemed as responsible enough to take that on.
> *Pam*: Yeah, definitely.

The classic professional word 'autonomy' seemed important to these groups. Some of the group had a sophisticated idea of what this meant in the healthcare setting:

> *MT*: And are nurses people who are autonomous?
> *Fred*: Not completely because they're also directed by the medical team on what's needed. You know, a nurse wouldn't just go off and take blood gases; there'd probably be some kind

of deterioration, the doctor would be called and the doctor would take the blood gases based on their clinical judgement. So they're more autonomous than we are but they're, you know, everybody's accountable to somebody at the end of the day. Somewhere along the line, you've got to be accountable to somebody.

Pam: Good answer, absolutely right.

The sensitivities about professional demarcation discussed in the opening part of this chapter did not seem to be shared by these groups:

MT: So what would be the difference between what you will be doing when you finish the course and what nurses are doing?

Les: I think we'll just be more working closely together, cause even in our jobs, we work quite closely with the nurses anyway, we're practically on their level; the only thing we don't give would be medication, so I think it's the support of where you're working, like you said, we've got quite a lot of support from our nurses and from our hospital ...

Pam: Yeah, I just don't understand why they wouldn't be support-ive like, you're all doing the same work; you're a team so you can all share the work together so why is that such a problem?

However at other moments members did not see the healthcare occupations as such a happy family:

Fred: I think it's the PIN number was mentioned earlier and there's a big thing about protecting your PIN number – the nurses have their registration – and I think that that's what they're afraid is under threat. I don't think it's a fact that they'll be sharing work – I mean a lot of nurses would be happy to share some of their workload, I'm fairly certain of that, I think it's the fact that their position as staff nurses, registered nurses looks to be uncertain in the future, certainly with the probable registration of associate practitioners coming later on.

How work is moved 'down' the hierarchy

As I said earlier, the classic view of healthcare work has been to see it as dominated by a single profession, medicine. From this viewpoint the 'paramedical' professions, such as nursing, represent both an opportunity and a threat for medicine. They are a threat because they could always take over aspects of medical work, i.e. threaten its dominance (in theory at least). However, they provide an attractive opportunity because they allow medicine to delegate particular tasks – let's say tasks that have become repetitive or low status – in a way that can enhance the status of the more highly specialised work that is left. But the situation is always ambiguous partly because the same task can transmute in the process of handing it down from one profession to another, i.e. it changes from 'so specialised only we can be trusted to do it' to 'actually quite routine so that we can allow you to do it while we return to the exciting core of our proper work'.

The NHS Institute for Improvement and Innovation says nurses spend less than 40% of their time on direct patient care, and some studies put the figure far lower. 'Hunting and gathering' to find equipment or linen, chasing test results and non-nursing tasks were all cited to us as ways in which nursing and midwifery capital is misused and underused.

Some research suggests practitioners do not always want to spend more time with service users, or are not encouraged to. The reasons include the structures in which they work, the perceived low status of essential care, the need to 'get the work done', and 'the stress of emotional labour'.

Source: Prime Minister's Commission 2010: 50

The classic discussion is of *delegation*, where the more powerful profession initiates the transfer of certain work to the less powerful group. However, more recently governments have intervened to open up previously restricted work to other occupations. Their motives may be either financial or to achieve other policy objectives which I discuss in Chapter 7.

Two initiatives, promoted by the government, rather than directly instigated by doctors are cases in point where the change did not go without opposition. Nurse prescribing was first piloted in a limited form in 1994 and gradually extended since then, particularly in 2000 in the NHS Plan (Department of Health 2000). Before this the 1968 Medicines Act restricted the legal right to prescribe medicines to doctors, dentists and veterinary surgeons, and this legal right was one of the defining powers of doctors. The nurse (and pharmacist) prescribing initiative was not universally welcomed by doctors. A *Lancet* editorial spoke of nurses being flattered and manipulated by politicians (Horton 2002) in an unconsidered policy, and some doctors spoke of the practice as dangerous. For example a letter to the BMJ from 2005 gives a good account of the objectors' position:

> The British Medical Association's opposition to extended prescribing by nurses and pharmacists deserves strong support by every member of the profession. Extended prescribing by inadequately qualified personnel is an idea spawned by politicians who basically have no understanding of medicine, and think that medical care might be provided more rapidly by fostering a huge increase in the number of individuals with the power to prescribe. This measure might meet the approval of administrators and accountants, who are also devoid of medical knowledge and experience but are keen to cut down on expenditure.
>
> BMJ (2005)

However, a survey conducted in 2008 found moderate levels of support from doctors for nurse prescribing, one of the perceived benefits being that it saved time on 'routine work' (Bradley and Nolan 2008). The second example is NHS Direct. This was launched in 1998 (Department of Health 1997), and its aim was to manage demand for more costly GP and emergency services. It is a telephone service staffed by nurses who work closely to computer-guided protocols. The government currently plans to replace it with a 'non-emergency' 111 telephone service. The service has been criticised by the BMA GPs committee as not cost-effective, though the government claimed that in 2008 it saved 1.7 million GP consultations and privately many doctors questioned the trustworthiness of nurses' diagnostic abilities, 'diagnosis' like prescribing, being a cornerstone of medical practice.

In more conventional cases of delegation, we might expect the process to go more smoothly. However while this may be largely true, it does not mean that the process is a simple one. We can look to two useful concepts to make sense of what is at stake in the deliberations on the borders between professions. One is the notion of the indeterminacy/technicality ratio in occupational work and the other is the idea of 'dirty work'. We could say that the activities of all occupations can be investigated and placed along a continuum from highly technical to highly indeterminate. Technically defined work consists of activities that could be set out in a book of instructions, while indeterminacy describes the formation of expert, possibly difficult to articulate, judgements which, according to this theory, can only be made by individuals with personal qualities and particular training and experience distinctive to those within a particular occupation. According to this theory the indeterminacy/technicality ratio, or 'I/T ratio', in professional work relative to other occupational work would be high.[11] The notion of 'dirty work' originates from the study of stigmatised jobs, work that society 'delegates' to certain groups who then become stigmatised by association with this work, at least in terms of that society's overt values. Those studying 'dirty work' have been interested in how members of such occupations manage their 'tainted' identity. Also, 'insofar

[11] This theory Jamous, H. and B. Peloille (1970). Professions or Self-Perpetuating System; Changes in the French University-Hospital System. *Professions and Professionalisation*. J. Jackson (ed). Cambridge, Cambridge University Press: 109–152, is not new, dating from 1970, but it is still widely referred to. See Atkinson, P., M. Reid, et al. (1977). 'Medical Mystique'. *Sociology of Work and Occupations* **4**(3): 243–280, Carmel, S. (2003). High Technology Medicine in Practice: The Organisation of Work in Intensive Care. *Faculty of Medicine*. London, University of London (London School of Hygiene & Tropical Medicine). Traynor, M. (2009). 'Indeterminacy and Technicality Revisited: How Medicine and Nursing Have Responded to the Evidence Based Movement'. *Sociology of Health & Illness* **31**(4): 494–507.

as every occupation carries with it a self-conception, a notion of personal dignity, then it is likely that some of the work that its members do may threaten this dignity' (Allen 2001, p. 12). It is possible that such forces are at work in the attempts to shift tasks from one occupational group to another, or within one occupation from one sub-group to another.

Behind both of these theories, and the great many others about professional work, is the understanding that professions, like countries perhaps, are constantly under some degree of threat, or potential threat, or at the very least theoretical threat, and have to constantly work to minimise that threat and advance their own interests proactively. As I said earlier, the 'borders' between the work or area of responsibility of different groups represent both threat and opportunity. The healthcare support worker quoted earlier understood this when saying nurses would not have a problem 'sharing their workload' but are nervous about the continuing value of their registered status in the face of the creation of new types of worker such as APs. The challenge that nurses and doctors have is to convince managers and politicians that they offer something to health care that the others do not have. If they were unsuccessful, the fear is that the profession would dwindle in numbers, in the rewards offered, the authority it can exercise and ultimately be consigned to history along with switchboard operators, carpet-beaters and barber-surgeons.

Davina Allen shows examples of nurses policing the boundary between nursing and support worker roles. She quotes from the training given – by nurses – in one of the hospitals she studies, to new HCAs:

> Nurse Manager [GRETA]: Right – you are there to *assist* the registered nurse. You're not there to do the registered nurses' job. You're there to *assist* [...] You will not be involved in assessing patients [...]. You are there to *assist* in the implementation of care. Assessing patients can be anything from admitting a patient to doing a bed-bath and looking at them. As a registered nurse I can assess the situation there and then ... I am assessing all the

time because that's what I have been trained to do ... Assessment is a very fine line and it makes it very difficult to explain to you what you can and can't do.

Allen (2001: 83).[12]

The nurse manager is going to great lengths to differentiate the work of qualified nurses from that of support staff and, we might say, rather crudely putting the assistants 'in their place'. As Allen points out, the nurse does this, apart from through her bullying style, by reference to the indeterminacy of nursing work and the relative technicality of the assistants' role. 'Assessment', according to her, is such a subtle art that it is difficult to even to talk about, certainly in formalised terms that support staff could understand. Support staff, by contrast, are employed to carry out the range of tasks, 'assist in the implementation of care', determined by registered nurses. In other words, the work pushed across the boundary between 'real' nursing work and the proper work of support workers is subtly (or not so subtly) devalued by recasting it as routine, to do with the implementation of a care which is devised by nurses as a result of their expert assessment. The recipients of this delegated work on the other hand, at least those who joined my focus groups, described their work as 'the actual main work' which the nurse could no longer do as she was burdened with managerial and administrative distractions. Elsewhere they described their approach as 'holistic' because they have the time to 'sit and have a chat' with patients in contrast to other workers. In other words, how individuals understand work can be completely different depending on their position.

Although managerialism and financial forces affect both boundaries, potentially driving work 'downwards', the boundary between medical and nursing work has a different character to that between

---

[12] Allen's work was conducted in the late 1990s. Many of the underlying issues have not changed but the role and training, albeit hugely varied, of today's healthcare support workers have moved on considerably from that of the healthcare assistants of the 1990s.

nurses and support workers. Because it is an organised profession, nursing can make broadly collective responses to medical tactics that support workers are unable to do at present. Much of this response has been deeply ambivalent but it centres around conceptions of professional identity and status. One way of understanding the dilemma would be to consider that nursing has from its early days wished for some of the prestige and power of medicine, so taking on previously medical roles has a powerful symbolic attraction, nurse prescribing being one example. Learning and becoming proficient in new complex technical skills may also be rewarding for many nurses. However, to be *delegated* a series of possibly unwanted tasks by medicine would not enhance nursing's professional self-image, so should be resisted. In fact some have said that the idea of being a 'mini-doctor' is anathema for nurses. The challenge therefore has been to translate as much cross border movement into forms or language that is more consistent with a desirable nursing identity. So, doctors may move work such as taking blood, administering intravenous medicines and ECG recordings to nurses. This could be understood as jettisoning routine tasks, or it could be described as an opportunity to provide holistic, efficient and patient-centred care, seamlessly and without the interruption of passing the patient to and fro between different professionals. Both, in a sense, could be true, but my argument is that when it comes to such boundary work, it is in the interests of medicine to understand and describe it one way, and for nursing to present it as another, and in fact it will come naturally to each group to do so. I have shown this process happening on the border between nursing work and the work of HCSWs, and it is similar here.

I take a final, amusing example of boundary work from Davina Allen's book. Doctors have passed on the flushing of central lines[13] to nurses. In order to signal that nurses were sufficiently skilled for

---

[13] Central venous access devices.

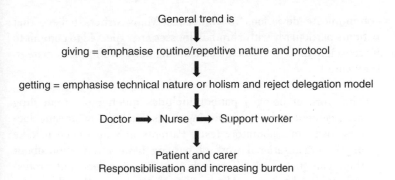

General trend is

⬇

giving = emphasise routine/repetitive nature and protocol

⬇

getting = emphasise technical nature or holism and reject delegation model

⬇

Doctor ➡ Nurse ➡ Support worker

⬇

Patient and carer
Responsibilisation and increasing burden

Figure 4.1 Handling healthcare work on the occupational borders

this delicate task, senior nurses developed an extensive range of training literature including test questions for nurses undertaking this work. However, on seeing the material a consultant surgeon commented that it was of such unnecessary complexity that he was unable to answer some of the test questions required and requested, with mocking irony, that as he was not qualified to handle this technology, the hospital abandon their use of central lines altogether (Figure 4.1).

The healthcare workers who don't get paid

Before closing this chapter on nursing's professional neighbours, I need to mention the changing role of patients and their carers. It is not new to point to the costs incurred by patients and carers in using health services. These are usually conceived as significant time and often financial, not to mention opportunity, costs. However recently we have seen technological 'advances' such as the development of telemedicine, coupled with a political shift entailing changing views of the behaviour expected of citizens. These changes can require patients or carers to take over ('self-manage') the work previously done by paid workers, such as monitoring and recording their condition. This places the onus on them to communicate deviations to clinicians. Many writers believe that patients particularly with chronic illnesses are expected to commit to increasingly time- and energy-consuming activities to participate in their care:

> The work of being a patient includes much more than drug management and self-monitoring. It also includes organising doctors' visits and laboratory tests. Patients may also need to take on the organisational work of passing basic information about their care between different healthcare providers and professionals... Advances in diagnosis and treatment thus have the paradoxical effect of adding incrementally to the work of being sick. Patients who cannot cope eventually experience iatrogenic outcomes and poorer quality of life.
>
> May, Montori et al. (2009)

In part this reflects an increasing 'responsibilisation' of patients, and the public generally, in health and other areas of life. This is usually presented positively as enabling and empowering patients and others to take control over their illness, life, etc. and counteract the bureaucratic or paternalistic features of large organisations like the UK NHS, and this could be true to a certain extent. But this definition presents another side of this contemporary and apparently benign tendency:

> [Responsibilisation is] a term developed in the governmentality[14] literature to refer to the process whereby subjects are rendered

---

[14] Governmentality has been defined as the organised practices through which subjects are governed, generally by governments, in an attempt to produce a citizen best suited to fulfil that government's policies. The concept has been particularly applied to the study of contemporary neoliberal governments that have emphasised notions of individual choice and responsibility. For one of the original articles about the concept, see Foucault, M. (1991). 'Governmentality', Trans. Rosi Braidotti and Revised by Colin Gordon. *The Foucault Effect: Studies in Governmentality*. G. Burchell, C. Gordon and P. Miller (eds). Chicago, IL, University of Chicago Press: 87–104.

individually responsible for a task which previously would have been the duty of another – usually a state agency – or would not have been recognized as a responsibility at all. The process is strongly associated with neoliberal political discourses, where it takes on the implication that the subject being responsibilised [!] has avoided this duty or the responsibility has been taken away from them in the welfare-state era and managed by an expert or government agency.

O'Malley (2009: 276)

This is a system-level issue which according to some writers is typically beyond the ability of individual health workers to address, but no consideration of the drive to reconfigure healthcare work would be complete without acknowledging the increasing role of unpaid carers and patients themselves. Like other aspects of this shifting work, it has to be viewed as ambiguous, with some positive outcomes but also unwelcome effects.

Summary

Who does what in healthcare changes over time. From a historical perspective, whole professions can disappear and new ones develop. On a more day-to-day level, work passes between occupations and there can be intense negotiation on the borders. Nursing is under pressure from the increasing use of APs to become more focussed on overseeing care while it is expected as a profession to maintain its close involvement with patients. But this is a permanent conundrum. Neither nurses nor support workers, nor any of the professions, can exist without the others. There is an interdependence. Many experienced nurses know that in order to do their job well, they have to be able to rely on support workers. When they are good and when all work together as a team, complementing each other's roles and skills, patient care can be good. But on a basic level nurses find it difficult to totally devolve care to HCSWs, as individualised patient care relies on nurses having a comprehensive knowledge of both the patient and the disease process that has brought them into the work environment. Experienced working nurses say that they cannot split themselves into many pieces, but they can use support workers to feed into their knowledge of patients and to support the overall care given.[15]

[15] Thanks to Linda Worpole, Clinical Nurse Specialist, Addenbrookes Hospital in Cambridge for her reflections which inform this summary.

5

'Evidence-Based Everything': The Use and Limits of Research

Today's healthcare practice and education set out to be 'evidence based'. Textbooks are peppered with the term. But it has not always been the case. This chapter explores the rise of the evidence based movement in medicine and nursing since approximately 1991 and its different flavour in the two professions. It reviews some of the arguments for and against the movement and in the process examines the much discussed notion of 'expert practice'. Some have claimed that evidence-based practice (EBP) can empower members of the healthcare team who have little status, and the movement was, in its early days, presented as a democratising and radical attack on authority-based health care where what the senior person liked was how care got delivered. The chapter argues that in the organisation and delivery of health care, improvements to the quality of leadership, communication or workload may have a larger effect on outcomes than 'implementing evidence'. This claim leads into the next chapter.

The two words 'evidence' and 'based', hinged by a hyphen, have crept into the English language and policy jargon over the last 20 years or so. Even politicians can be heard using the term to raise support for some course of action they are trying to promote. Like the most successful social movements, the once provocative arguments of a small group mainly of epidemiologists that gave rise to 'evidence-based medicine' (EBM) and its interdisciplinary variant 'evidence-based practice' now sound like common sense.

From what you have seen in care settings, how have decisions about care been made? It may often be difficult to tell, and it can even be difficult to detect when a decision has been made. The usual assumption is that health care is the sum of a series of clinical events involving diagnosis of an individual patient's illness followed by treatment and hopefully some kind of recovery. However the influences on actual care and treatment delivered in hospitals and community settings, including the administrative arrangements that surround and support this, sometimes defy unravelling. A recent report (Wise 2012) which found that outcomes in the NHS are worse for patients admitted at the weekend rather than during the week gives a clue that there are many factors that influence care. Perhaps the following have an influence on how and what care is delivered to any individual patient: which part of the service they come in contact with and which speciality, the seniority and experience of the individual who first assesses them, how busy or pressured the service is, whether there is timely access to diagnostic services, whether their notes get lost or not, the quality of overall management, the quality of communication between different parts of the service and between different professionals, the quality of communication between professionals and the patient. If this is true, then the common or early focus of EBP on the moment of the clinician's decision making around a particular clinical intervention moves slightly away from centre stage.

There are a huge number of books, articles and websites devoted to defining and promoting EBP in nursing. My aim in this chapter is not to provide more information or to exhort the reader to try harder to understand or implement it. My aim, in line with the other chapters in this book, is to fill in the context and background to the rise of EBP and to summarise, in a broadly even-handed way, the fierce arguments that have been made for and against it. As I have repeated, the issues facing nurses and others in today's health care are often presented as technical problems, but all come already with political and professional contexts and forces built in. If we are not aware of these, then we are practising (and learning) like automata, not sophisticated people. And if we want to influence health care, or even simply survive in it, we need to have a sophisticated understanding of what is going on.

Evidence-based medicine emerged as a piece of terminology in the early 1990s. The movement tells its own story about the style of practice that it set out to replace and about its benefits, so that now it is difficult to remember what health care was like before it gained such prominence. What is not so easy to forget is the evangelical force and style with which it was promoted and the controversy that it engendered among practitioners. By evangelical I mean a style of argument, adopted by some religious groups, with three characteristic stages: first, *even though it might seem otherwise* the present situation is seriously problematic; second, our group's solution defines the field in such a way that it is the only significant solution so if you are not for us, you are part of the problem; third, you can and you must be converted to our way of thinking and your life will radically change, then you can join in the work to convert others. Of course EBM promoters are not the only group that can be described in this way but you can see that it is a particularly uncompromising type of argument. EBM arose within a speciality of medicine, clinical epidemiology, and while it was still a cause of angry letters to medical editors, it was launched into nursing where, though not without its opponents, it was accepted rather more eagerly. Though it raised particular issues for nursing, it promised what the profession constantly craves – legitimacy.

The phenomenon of the rise of the evidence-based movement is fascinating for a number of reasons: we can think about how the movement might represent a challenge to conventional ideas of professional work and expertise, it tells us something about society's ideas concerning risk and it also tells us something about the relationship between policy makers, managers and clinicians. I plan to spend this chapter exploring what EBM and EBP might mean for practising nurses. But first it is important to understand where the idea came from and what enabled it to develop and gain the dominance that it has in a surprisingly short time.

Why did evidence-based practice catch on?

In March 1988, responding to a decline in the standing of UK science and technology, the House of Lords Select Committee on Science and Technology investigated 'Priorities in Medical Research'. The Committee reported that 'the NHS was run with little awareness of the needs of research or what it had to offer' (House of Lords Select Committee on Science and Technology 1988). The inquiry resulted in the formation of the NHS's first research and development (R&D) strategy, launched in 1991, astonishingly over 40 years since the service's foundation.

> The prime objective [of the strategy] is to see that R&D becomes an integral part of health care so that clinicians, managers and other staff find it *natural* to rely on the results of research in their day-to-day decision making and longer term strategic planning. Strongly held views based on belief rather than sound information still exert too much influence in health care.
>
> (My emphasis) (Department of Health 1991)

The Evidence-Based Medicine movement emerged and took hold in the United Kingdom alongside the rise of research promotion in the Department of Health and the NHS. For better or worse, it quickly became associated with a number of charismatic figures (Smith 1991). The most notable was David Sackett originally from McMaster University in Canada in North America's first clinical epidemiology department.

Funding was found for organisations such as the Centre for Reviews and Dissemination based in York, United Kingdom and the Cochrane Collaboration in Oxford, United Kingdom, named after Scottish clinician Archie Cochrane, advocate of the randomised controlled trial (RCT), to be set up specifically to commission or carry out systematic reviews of suitable research and to disseminate much-needed 'evidence' to clinicians and managers. A key feature of the EBM movement was that it made no bones that the RCT and the systematic review of these trials were to be understood as the 'gold standard' of research evidence, a well-conducted experiment being considered the best way of determining the effectiveness of particular interventions – in theory at least. The Cochrane Collaboration became a global resource of systematic reviews, contributed to by clinicians and reviewers around the world. The movement focussed on a characteristic trinity of concerns: critical appraisal (a systematic way of evaluating the quality of research papers), compiling systematic reviews (a similar highly formalised way of assessing quality and combining the findings of a number of high quality studies) and the implementation of suitable research findings (which EBM advocates came to realise was possibly the most difficult challenge of the whole process) (Lomas 1993).

Because the emphasis on research-mindedness emerged in the context of an ever sharpening focus on healthcare costs and cost-effectiveness (Redmayne 1995), and of increasing managerial scrutiny of health care (Harrison and Pollitt 1994; Traynor 1996), which I discuss in other chapters, many disgruntled clinicians thought it represented a significant threat to medical autonomy. In reality EBM was, partly, an attempt to forestall such a challenge and establish control over research and the useful managerial information it could provide within the medical profession and not outside it.

EBM and its supporters were often controversial, and fierce debates started to appear in the pages of UK medical journals from 1991 in the form of letters, editorials and other articles. Criticism focussed both on the 'style' of the movement which some found unacceptably evangelical, as I mentioned. For example, a Lancet editorial from 1995 describes the movement's 'strident insistence' and promotion of a 'new orthodoxy' as having risked antagonising doctors (Horton 1995). Others detected the presence of a 'backlash' against the movement produced by 'the fears of some clinicians that [its] concepts threaten the art of patient care' (Naylor 1995). I come back to the idea that there is an 'art' of medical or nursing practice.

Perhaps what caused the trouble was that the movement challenged a powerful and deeply entrenched medical establishment by questioning the fundamental principle of individual clinical autonomy. Looking back in an interview on TVO, a public television broadcaster in Ontario, Canada (currently available at http://www.youtube.com/watch?v=Nbd–s2dFY0), recorded in 2009, David Sackett acknowledges that EBM divided the medical establishment along the lines of 'the old guys' and 'the young guys'. For him, the techniques of EBM provided the ammunition and the confidence for junior medics to challenge senior figures about their un-evidence-based and possibly idiosyncratic preferences. Elsewhere he wrote about the predicament of medical students and junior doctors who have, he says, to carry out the orders of their consultants, unaware of whether:

> the advice received from the experts is authoritative (evidence-based ...) or merely authoritarian (opinion-based, resulting from pride and prejudice).
>
> Sackett (2000: 5)

Sackett crossed the Atlantic to work in the university city of Oxford as foundation Director of the NHS R&D Centre for Evidence-Based Medicine and Consultant on the Medical Service at the John Radcliffe Hospital, and it is not difficult to imagine that his north American style, along with his background in epidemiology (hitherto a relatively low status area of medicine) did not endear him to the more establishment end of the Oxford medical world.

In 1996 five high profile promoters of EBM published a letter in the BMJ under the heading 'Evidence based medicine: what it is and what it isn't' (Sackett, Rosenberg et al. 1996). What had started out as a direct confrontation to medical expertise was carefully redrawn as a judicious mixture of 'clinical expertise and the best available external evidence' (Sackett, Rosenberg et al. 1996: 71). It was simply what 'good doctors' do.

Evidence and the 'risk' society

EBP, in many ways, was a child of its time. It emerged during a period preoccupied with a) risk, b) ambivalence about the status and role of experts (the inquiry into the deaths of babies in the UK Bristol Royal Infirmary (Kennedy and Bristol Royal Infirmary 2000) provided a focus for those who wished to bring clinicians under sharper scrutiny), and c) concerned with effectiveness, the following of procedures, and the power of the consumer (Trinder 2000). EBP deals with all of these concerns, relates them to one another, redefines some and rolls them up into well-integrated package. If sociologist Anthony Giddens and other commentators were right when they claimed that there was a crisis of belief in science and expertise, we might ask, 'why has a movement so firmly based in science and rationality been so successful', particularly at a time when social science had turned away from quests for an unchanging or a unified body of knowledge? The response of EBM to this mood of scepticism has been what Giddens termed 'sustained optimism' in the possibility that rational thought and technology can provide solutions to our problems of insecurity (Giddens 1990). EBP demands that a much more rigorous and systematic science be applied by practitioners, but it is not the science of grand theory and new discovery, rather it is an attempt to keep harm at bay, a defensiveness which some have argued has become characteristic of contemporary science (Beck 1992).

Second to risk as an important contextual factor is the rise of managerialism and the imperative of transparency within the public sector. These forces rose to prominence partly as mechanisms of financial control, but partly as an ideological challenge to the power of established professions (see Chapter 7). With the public's trust in professionals waning and the New Right's political challenge, it seemed that transparent, impersonal *procedures*, like those involved in audit, were potentially more trustworthy as the basis of national health care than the authority of experts. According to one writer, 'the core of evidence-based practice is its procedures rather than its outputs' (Trinder 2000: 9). In only a few years the Cochrane Collaboration produced a huge array of procedures, checklists and guidelines. But EBP was also a challenge to managerialism and managers rather than simply a collusion because managerialism had focussed, up to then, on economy and efficiency but not on effectiveness.

EBP, then, represented an attempt to establish professionally defined effectiveness.

The final part of the context was the rise of information technology. The movement itself could not have developed as it did without electronic databases and the Internet for two reasons. First, they enable the international Cochrane Collaboration to function, but second and perhaps ironically, one of the key pillars of the movement is its argument that the individual practitioner cannot keep up to date with proliferating medical information which is itself partly a result of burgeoning IT capabilities.

Nursing and evidence

The promotion of EBP in nursing emerged in the wake of a long-standing promotion of research-mindedness in the profession, with the often repeated claim that much nursing practice was based on 'traditions, myths and rituals' (Walsh and Ford 1989). As I have mentioned before, the quest for legitimacy and standing has been a strong force in nursing since its appearance, and new movements, as they arise in health care, are usually approached by nursing as opportunities to further its own interests. (See Chapter 8 for the Chief Nursing Officer's opinion on policy opportunism.)

In London, in 1997, as a signal of professional backing, the journal *Evidence Based Nursing* was launched jointly by the BMJ and the Royal College of Nursing Publishing Company. Nursing quickly gained its own Centre for Evidence Based Nursing at the University of York in the United Kingdom. In Australia, the Joanna Briggs Institute for Evidence Based Nursing and Midwifery, based in Adelaide, was established in 1996, and many centres worldwide now identify with evidence-based nursing and run workshops on the topic. In short, the profession embraced the notion. I now talk about the tensions on the way.

Responses from nursing: 'Nurses care'

The challenge of EBP represented a dilemma for nursing. On the one hand, many nurse leaders have gone to considerable lengths to convince policy makers, managers and others that nursing is science-based activity, rather than a fundamentally morally based activity (Reverby 1987; ICN 1996; Thompson 1997). On the other hand, some nurses have felt uncomfortable about drawing on what they see as the same model of science (and research) as that taken up by doctors to do this (Cullum 1997) because it threatens an ideology, discussed in Chapter 4, where nursing is presented as a kind of antithesis to medicine ('doctors cure, nurses care'). In particular, many nursing writers have written critically about the emphasis on the RCT which EBP continually claims as the 'gold standard' of evidence. Their critiques often concern issues that practitioners of RCTs are well aware of themselves, for example the relevance of research findings from studies of carefully vetted and homogenised participants to 'real-life' clinicians facing patients with multiple morbidities (Seers 1997).

While there has been official acceptance and promotion of EBP in nursing, as in medicine, many influential figures in academic nursing have vigorously questioned it. John Paley has summarised the main objections to EBP by nurses (Paley 2006), and he has little time for their attempts to defend the traditional professional concepts of expertise and indeterminate clinical judgement against the challenge of EBP. Some defences of this view of expertise claim that standard accounts of EBP imply an overly narrow view of evidence, and that a more inclusive concept incorporating some degree of indeterminacy should be adopted. Others claim that statistical generalisations cannot be applied non-problematically to individual patients in specific contexts, and that this is why we need clinical judgement. As a response to the first argument, Paley mounts a fierce challenge to indeterminacy, arguing that the so-called ways of knowing, promoted by the champions of professional experience-based tacit knowledge, could more accurately be described as 'ways of coming to believe'. This is because, he argues, they fail to incorporate any procedure that is capable of identifying and eliminating error and in cases where this has been done, tacit knowledge has been found wanting in terms of delivering the best judgement. In Chapter 4 I introduced the terms 'indeterminacy' and 'technicality' as they apply to professional work. It might not surprise you to find the language of indeterminacy relied n by some of those criticising EBP. A leading academic mental health nurse for example has claimed that:

'The notion that we should or perhaps even could base our practice on 'generalisable evidence' demolishes our traditional practice. Such worldviews urge us to swap our ideas of crafting care around the unique complexity of the individual, for a generalisation about what worked for most people in a study'.
(Barker 2000: 332, cited in Paley 2006: 82)

Passages like this present an appealing and nostalgic picture of nursing and a harsh picture of EBP standing against nursing's valuable traditions. Similar arguments can be found in the letters pages of nursing periodicals from mental health nurses. This speciality is characterised by polarised views of practice with long-running debates between the champions of highly contextual approaches to practice, such as the writer above, and those promoting the importance of practice focussed on objective outcome measures (Barker 2000; Gournay 2000). Other critiques of EBP described by Paley feature the defence of a valued ideal version of healthcare practice:

EBP involves the neglect of 'holistic treatments tailored to individual patients, in favour of common approaches drawn inappropriately from aggregated data'.
(Kitson 2002: 179, cited in Paley 2006: 86)

By contrast, many nursing writers (sometimes the same writers in different contexts) looked to EBP to provide a similar kind of professional legitimacy as nursing theories had appeared to offer 30 years before, arguing that well-articulated evidence claims could 'demonstrate the value of nursing' (Kitson 1997; McClarey and Duff 1997).

In summary, the emergence of the evidence-based movement brought to a focus tensions within medicine and nursing around representations of both as individually focussed clinical encounters yet as embodying some of the disinterestedness of scientific activities.

> Three questions about decisions:
>
> 'Evidence-based nursing can be defined as the application of valid, relevant, research-based information in nurse decision making' (Cullum, Ciliska et al. 2008, p. 2). Given the difficulty sometimes in locating the actual site of decision making, identify an occasion from your experience in healthcare settings when a course of action regarding a patient was discussed and a decision arrived at. Make a list, or a diagram, of the following:
>
> 1. What was that setting and who was involved, e.g. was it a single nurse in front of a computer, a multidisciplinary meeting, etc.?
> 2. What resources were mentioned, e.g. local guidelines or policies, a research article, a story, an individual (a research nurse or a clinical librarian), expressed patient wishes, expressed or assumed clinician preferences?
> 3. What was the process, e.g. was it in the form of a discussion or instruction, were there presentations, if so how were they discussed, how were the different sources of information valued by participants?
>
> For an article about the complexity of knowledge management and (attempts at) evidence-based decision making, see Gabbay, Le May et al. 2003. This article contrasts the conventional neat diagram of the evidence-based approach, featuring seven identical linked boxes, with a diagram representing the knowledge behaviour exhibited at a meeting observed by the researchers designed to evaluate and put evidence into practice. In Gabbay and colleagues' diagram there are curved lines and chaotic text with no discernible direction of motion. One reviewer of the article described this figure as 'a total mess'. The authors replied, 'Yes, that's exactly right'.

Can evidence-based practice empower nurses (and others)?

When EBM first appeared it was presented as a direct challenge to a medical expertise which some felt was based too much on hierarchy and power and not enough on science. David Sackett wrote light-heartedly but no less provocatively:

> [UK] house officers, up to 75% of whom haven't read anything about the problems presented by their patients in the previous week, are being taught by senior consultants, up to 40% of whom haven't read anything either!
>
> Sackett (1997: 8)

His handbook *Evidence-Based Medicine: How to Practice and Teach EBM* makes a link with the history of the French Revolution and the European Enlightenment when legendary French clinicians like Pierre Louis 'rejected the pronouncements of authorities and sought the truth in systematic observation of patients' (Sackett 2000: 2). The argument goes, if evidence can become the new currency in health care then any clinician conscientious enough to spend time in a library (or, increasingly, in front of a computer) and armed with some simple techniques can have a say. Of course as we all know the powerful, even if they exercise their power illegitimately, find ways of holding on to it, nevertheless this aspect of the EB argument seems to have something in it. Research (not RCTs) does seem to indicate that sometimes nurses feel they can have input into clinical decisions if they can refer to research to support their suggestions.

In focus groups I carried out in 2008 with qualified nurses attending post-qualifying courses at my university, some nurses talked about how they used evidence to challenge their employer's current policies and could overrule doctors' instructions about particular practice by applying the 'trump card' of research evidence:

> *Health Visitor*: I had to do a report on a case that went to a child protection meeting [...] so I got a much bigger knowledge of that than [I had before]. I had to do a report on this child which contained stuff that went back to various NICE reports, guidelines and technology assessment which I knew the trust doesn't actually implement but in doing that it brought to the attention of the managers further up that we could actually be doing some of

the things we're not doing so it has changed practice and they are looking at getting some equipment and stuff.

Children's Nurse: ... The doctors [...] they have like left a cannula in too long and research says if its longer than 24 hours you should take it out. Its 72 hours [...] you know [...]. But still, and I would talk straight to them like 'I'm removing this because blah blah blah' and they would say 'oh no – but', I'd say 'no BUT'. So they say 'ok, take it out'. So [its] because I have that confidence and even though I'm newly qualified.

How often this kind of challenge happens is hard to know, and there is plenty of research that seems to suggest that actual uptake of research by nurses (however that is defined and measured) is relatively low (Hicks, Hennessy et al. 1996; McKenna, Ashton et al. 2004; Hek and Shaw 2006). Many organisations including professional bodies, agencies such as NICE (The National Institute for Health and Clinical Excellence) and individual NHS organisations issue guidelines for practitioners which are (usually) attempts to distil the findings of research on particular treatments and topics into summaries of best practice. Although sometimes practitioners are sceptical about how useful these are, they could be one way that clinicians 'put research into practice' without necessarily realising it.

A final word about EBP

Operating the National Health Service is complex. A huge number of factors have to be right for the system to work well. Some of these are to do with infrastructure and investment, some to do with workforce, the changing needs of a population, treatments and drugs available, computer systems, procurement of supplies and many other details. All of these factors depend on knowledge. Nevertheless the challenges in any particular area may not be primarily to do with lack of knowledge or uncertainty. They may be more to do with having managers with the right skills, adequate budget, the right people contributing to policy and decision making, the balance of political forces, and the motivation of staff. In other words in many of these areas, the best thing to do may already be clear. The difficulty may be making it happen. Apart from this, there will still be a great many areas where there is uncertainty and where additional knowledge could improve some aspect of services. Given the complexity of the organisation and running of the service, the types of uncertainty that exist and the types of knowledge needed will be extremely varied. Much of the knowledge needed will already exist somewhere, and the challenge will be sourcing and using it. For the rest, in the words of the credit card advertisement, there's research. So, although having investment in R&D and staff who are concerned with asking questions about improving services is absolutely vital, the research imperative has got to be understood in context. Given the complexity of the service, the types of research question that could be posed will be wide-ranging. We could group the types of question in this way: those concerning workforce configuration, recruitment, management and training; those investigating patient experience and preference; and those examining the effectiveness of interventions. It is chiefly in this last group of questions where the procedures of EBP are relevant and helpful. Research investigating the sometimes difficult relationship between managers and clinicians, for example, would be difficult to fit into the typical structures of EBP questions. But it is clear that for the good running of the service, these research questions need to be asked. In other words, the scope of EBP has particular parameters. The language used by many promoting EBP among clinicians does not tend to include these disclaimers, and for those new to research it sometimes appears that EBP documents are making general statements about research rather than specific ones. A well-used example is the 'hierarchy of evidence' often presented in EBP literature that features randomised trials at or near the top, and other research designs lower down. This does not make sense, for example, for questions such as the one above.[1] Nor would popular

---

[1] Some EBP advocates would disagree, arguing that nearly any area of uncertainty can be used as the basis for a randomised experiment of some kind.

EBP frameworks for asking questions such as 'PICO' (Patient [or population or problem], intervention, comparison and outcome).

The National Institute for Health Research

Earlier, I mentioned the NHS's first R&D strategy. Since 1991 the strategy, priorities and funding streams have developed. But from the point of view of those who work in healthcare research, its continued existence and funding is welcome. Currently there are five major research streams funded by NIHR: Research for Patient Benefit (RfPB) Programme, Invention for Innovation (i4i) Programme, Public Health Research (PHR) Programme, Health Services and Delivery Research Programme and Efficacy and Mechanism Evaluation (EME) Programme.

A body of nursing research?

For decades nurses involved in research have been urged by research leaders to concentrate their efforts on building a body of definitive research that establishes the effectiveness of nursing interventions, i.e. concentrate on the last group of questions above – or at least this call has been understood in this way. The argument has been that too much research done by nurses is exploratory, driven by individual interest and parochial, and because of this there is no sense that the profession is going forward in research terms. I want to end this chapter with an attempt to clarify this conundrum. We could argue that one feature of good research is that it provides knowledge that might be useful for situations and settings different to that in which the research was carried out. This is part of what is meant by building a body of research. To do this researchers typically attend to issues of sampling (Are my participants in some way representative of others? Is the sample big enough?) and overall quality and rigour. But there are other additional requirements for ensuring wider and more long-lasting usefulness. These include asking important and non-parochial questions (or understanding local concerns as instances of more general questions), and interpreting findings within some established theoretical context and thereby making some contribution to that theoretical context and debate. Given the multitude of health service research questions that nurses are well placed to ask, the theoretical, or disciplinary, context and potential contribution of that research will also be varied. For certain questions a biomedical approach, from which EBP developed, is appropriate, and for others the typical concerns, tools and theories developed in the social sciences are right.[2] Sometimes the call to develop a body of knowledge about nursing is heard as a call for hypothesis-testing biomedical style research. This is needed but so is research starting from and contributing to other fields of knowledge. For example, the previous chapter set out what is known from research about professional work, the interactions of professions with each other and with the state, and is built on concepts, such as 'dominance' or 'closure' developed within that field. This is a large and important area of research, relevant to practising nurses, but none of it involves clinical trials. What is important is the scope and ambition of research undertaken by nurses not so much whether it focuses on evaluating a nursing clinical intervention.

---

[2] Social scientists have studied how organisations work, how people communicate with each other, how national policy is developed and how people experience chronic illness. The classic fields of social science include anthropology, economics, history, political science, psychology and sociology.

6

The Mystery of Poor Care: Why?

When nurses apparently fail to care, it is big news. It deeply unsettles the picture that we like to think the public has of nursing and that the profession works hard to promote of nurses' work as fundamentally about caring. This chapter discusses the way that so-called poor performance is managed within the National Health Service (NHS) and approached by the Nursing and Midwifery Council (NMC). It reviews some of the research and other writing about these failures to care. Some of this writing offers explanations about how certain professional cultures, for example a culture of deference to medicine or deep-seated powerlessness, make collusion in poor or dangerous practice more likely. The research includes recent work that investigates the possibility that there is a streak in nursing culture where a complaint of victimhood delivers a certain kind of satisfaction, and offers an alternative to taking up power to change – or leaving altogether. I propose that to some extent health sys tems rely on this collective stance of powerlessness, for example the willingness to continue to work in environments that others would find unacceptable and reluctance to leave, for their continued functioning.

Recently I went to the Nursing Standard Nurse of the Year Awards in London. It's an event with high production values: light shows, smoke machines, loud music, a high profile media presenter (former newsreader Angela Rippon when I went) and even massive indoor fireworks at the end. The magazine asks readers for nominations of outstanding nurses, and then a panel of judges picks the best. Video vignettes of the work of the shortlisted nurses are shown before they come on stage to receive their award and huge applause. The purpose of the event has always been to celebrate and publicise what is good about nursing and individual nurses. Everyone present enjoys an evening of glamour and good food. By coincidence, the year I attended, the evening fell shortly after yet another blistering attack on poor quality nursing in the media. This time it was the columnist Christina Patterson on Radio 4's *Four Thought: Care to Be a Nurse?*[1] Christina who had breast cancer and then a reoccurrence told in unsparing detail about her two stays in hospital. During both she was dealt with by cruel – that was the word she used – nurses. She ended by saying that there may be any number of structural explanations for the puzzle that people go into an apparently caring profession only to behave in a far from caring way, but she pointed to a fundamental personal responsibility. Each nurse, she said, had a decision to make either to be cruel or to be kind, and if they did not like the work they could leave. Her harrowing personal account came amid other media reports including secretly filmed experiences of vulnerable patients in hospitals and care homes in the United Kingdom at the hands of shockingly uncaring nurses and care assistants.

At Nurse of the Year, awareness of this kind of negative publicity was everywhere. Both Peter Carter, General Secretary of the RCN, and Christine Beasley, Chief Nurse for England, spoke about it with concern in their addresses. So did Angela Rippon. She talked about the 'bad apples' in nursing, as many people do. However, I felt there was something desperate this year to blow away these disturbing images of the profession. Was the music louder than ever before? Had there ever been such enormous fireworks at the climax of the show? And at the end of the evening when the year's Nurse of the Year announced to the audience that she was proud to be a nurse, the entire audience shot to its feet in a standing ovation. Angela repeated this triumphant phrase once the applause had died down a little calling out 'and you should be proud to be a great

---

[1] The programme has been available on the BBC website at http://www.bbc.co.uk/iplayer/episode/b010mrzt/Four_Thought_Series_2_Care_to_be_a_nurse/.

profession'. However, despite all this celebration the question of why some nurses appear to act in uncaring and sometimes even cruel ways towards their patients was left unaddressed. It is this difficult topic that I want to discuss in this chapter.

I start by describing the spectrum of nursing 'poor performance', how this has been defined and the often inadequate way that it has been dealt with in the NHS.[2]

Nurses and midwives make up the largest clinical group in the UK NHS and because of their close and constant interaction with patients they have great potential to influence patient experience and outcomes. Also, partly as a result of health policy over the last 12 years, their field of responsibility has been growing, now including, for example, the power to prescribe medicines. Nurses also manage various services, often for the chronically ill, and run technical investigative provision such as endoscopy. As is the case with the other professional groups involved in health care, the vast majority of nurses and midwives are highly skilled and conscientious practitioners, and the number of those who represent what might be termed 'a cause for concern' appears to be extremely small. As I mentioned in Chapter 3, the NMC acts as the police for the profession. Individuals who for example commit a criminal offence that may have no direct link to their nursing work, face having their name removed from the Register and hence are prohibited from working as a nurse or midwife. When a nurse or midwife is reported to the NMC, the Council first tries to determine whether there is a case to answer and if there is, starts an investigation. Those at the receiving end of NMC investigations amount to between 0.2% and 0.3% of nurses (Nursing and Midwifery Council 2009, 2011). Nevertheless,

---

[2] This is based on a scoping study that I carried out for the National Clinical Advisory Service (NCAS) with colleagues. See Stone, K., Traynor, M., Gould, D. and Maben, J. (2011). The management of poor performance in nursing and midwifery: A Case for Concern. *Journal of Nursing Management* DOI: 10.1111/j.1365-2834.2011.01219.x. NCAS was set up in April 2001 (as the National Clinical Assessment Authority) in response to a number of financially and personally damaging suspensions of senior doctors.

unacceptable or dangerous practice, whether through lack of training or poor support, illness, alcoholism, lack of motivation or ill-intent has potentially grave consequences. And as the stream of highly publicised cases emphasises, nurses are charged to care for some of the most vulnerable in society such as children, those with learning difficulties and the elderly. Some nurses and midwives work alone with high degrees of decision-making autonomy and less access to professional development and the scrutiny of colleagues. There are calls for nurses' roles to expand further and for an increased presence in community – and hence potentially isolated – settings. For all these reasons, the way that poor performance is managed is an important issue for the profession, for the health service and, of course, for patients and the public.

NCAS (see footnote to previous page) defined performance concerns as: 'any aspects of a practitioner's performance or conduct which:

- pose a threat or potential threat to patient safety;
- expose services to financial or other substantial risk;
- undermine the reputation or efficiency of services in some significant way;
- are outside acceptable practice guidelines and standards'.

National Clinical Assessment Service (2010: 2)

However, until I started to look into the subject of poor performance in nursing and medicine, I had no idea how complex and murky the topic was. The crucial part of the story is that in any particular case prior to the involvement of the NMC, the GMC (General Medical Council) for doctors, or the other health professions' own regulators, a clinician about whom there are concerns experiences his or her employer's disciplinary procedures.

The story in the literature goes something like this: The NHS is wasting huge amounts of money paying the salaries of, often, senior doctors who are suspended on full pay while protracted investigations into some aspect of their conduct are carried out. Sometimes these doctors can be on 'gardening leave' for years, while their employer shells out for a replacement and investigations, which can escalate to different levels, move at a glacial pace. If this was not bad enough, there is the huge personal impact of being escorted off the premises, often without warning or full explanation with the stern caution not to attempt to contact any colleagues which would be seen as an attempt to 'tamper with witnesses'.

As some of the researchers whose work I present later have noted, these procedures often happen completely out of the eye of external scrutiny, have been described as 'quasi-official', and it is not unusual for employees who are subsequently dismissed to be required by their ex-employer to sign an agreement not to make disclosures about the matter in public. However, many of these clinicians are not, ultimately, given the sack but are suspended from work pending some kind of investigation into their activities. According to the Arbitration Conciliation and Advisory Service (ACAS), suspension is 'a neutral act'. According to every guidance document from the Department of Health, it is a last resort to be used only when patient safety is threatened (Department of Health and National Patient Safety Agency 2006; National Clinical Assessment Service 2010). According to those who have been suspended however, it is a totally devastating act that can lead to financial collapse and mental breakdown. But surely, if a nurse or midwife has, for example, shown a serious lack of clinical skill or judgement that has put patients at risk, or has behaved inappropriately toward them, then it is only right that this individual is removed from causing more harm, pending a careful decision about further action.

Unfortunately, it is not that simple. My first tentative searches into the topic revealed a large amount of dissatisfaction and vitriol posted on Internet sites by aggrieved victims of NHS suspension. After my research was published I began to receive in the post anonymous accounts of grievances that individual nurses have expressed with their employers and the NMC. It seems, according to many of these voices, that among the suspended are those who describe themselves as whistleblowers who have got on the wrong side of managers or colleagues because of their refusal to be silent about poor care. These individuals see themselves as innocent victims of corrupt and collusive systems which are trying to silence them. So, we have a complete reversal of the assumption that the suspended represent the 'bad apples' of the profession. Among the suspended could be the very nurses and midwives who have the highest personal standards. Some suspensions seem bizarre such as the case of the 'crouton surgeon', Terence Hope, consultant neurosurgeon at Queen's Medical Centre in Nottingham, who was sent home following 'allegations about his personal conduct', that is, claims that he had taken a second portion of soup from the staff canteen without paying. An article in the Guardian reported, 'A BMA spokesman said suspensions should be made only for cases of gross misconduct, not claims that a surgeon failed to pay for a £1.03 bowl of soup' (Carvel 2004). Other suspensions and disciplinary procedures appear more complex and even sinister. The group Campaign Against Unnecessary Suspensions & Exclusions in the NHS keeps a catalogue of accounts of suspensions from the point of view of the suspended individual and provides links to a number of reports on the subject at http://www.suspension-nhs.org/.

The NMC code of practice states that as a nurse or midwife, you: 'must act without delay if you believe that you, a colleague or anyone else may be putting someone at risk'. However, it seems that it is not unusual for no action to be taken or at least no feedback to be given about action taken after such 'whistleblowing'. In one piece of research with nurses and consultants in a UK NHS trust (Firth-Cozens, Firth et al. 2003), 42% of nurses (144) reported they would consider whistleblowing poor practice with 63% (90) having gone ahead with it. The reasons for reporting poor performance were mainly poor clinical practice and poor behaviour and patient abuse. Of the 70 nurses who answered a question on repercussions of reporting poor performance, 51% (36) stated they had not suffered negative consequences as a result of reporting, 27% said that they had suffered victimisation by colleagues as a consequence of reporting and 13% said nothing had happened. Nevertheless, almost all nurses stated they would whistleblow again. The nurses who did not whistleblow (198) said that the claim was often 'impossible to prove', they were 'not sure if they were right' or did not like the idea of 'hurting a colleague' (p. 334). The researchers noted that in many cases people who have reported poor performance find that nothing is done as a result. The work also highlighted the difference in attitudes between nurses and doctors stating: 'The most striking difference in the data is that doctors are so much less likely than nurses to perceive and to report poor behaviour or abuse of patients and staff' (p. 335). Other research has suggested that student nurses (Bellefontaine 2009) and midwives (Currie and Richens 2009) are reluctant to report poor practice for fear of being labelled troublemaker or of repercussions.

A doctor who described herself as 'the whistleblower for Ward 87 City General Hospital, North Staffordshire NHS Trust' claims on a number of Internet sites (for example http://sites.google.com/site/ward87whistleblower/) that her complaints about standards of care resulted in an investigation into her conduct and character by the GMC which even questioned her own mental health. More well known is the case of nurse Margaret Haywood who was involved in a BBC documentary about poor care and secretly filmed the neglect of elderly patients at Royal County Sussex Hospital during 2004 (BBC Panorama 2009). She claimed managers had taken no notice when she had expressed concerns. She was struck off by the NMC in 2008 for misconduct on the grounds that she had breached patient confidentiality but later reinstated, apparently after an intervention from the RCN which had begun legal action, this reversal pointing to how the meaning of 'the code' is, at the end of the day, decided socially and consensually rather than in an objective way. Margaret Haywood went on to receive the patients' favourite award at the Nursing Standard Nurse of the Year awards in 2009.

The nursing and local press reports a steady stream of similar stories of nurses and others, apparently disciplined after speaking out about poor care. The problem with many of these stories is that they are likely to mask a complex situation with their simplistic labels. The individual lauded by the press as brave whistleblower may be arrogant, uncooperative and impossible to work with from the point of view of their colleagues or managers. The person charged by a trust management or the NMC's solicitors as arrogant, uncooperative and impossible to work with (as background to some misconduct case for example), may be someone who refuses to collude in a culture of mediocrity or actual harm. It has been my impression from attendance at a small number of NMC fitness to practise hearings and from reading the accounts of the 'charges' on the regulator's website (http://www.nmc-uk.org/Hearings/Hearings-and-outcomes/) that the incident that has lead to the investigation is often the culmination of a series of lesser problems none of which on its own has justified an individual being reported, (but then neither has possibly remedial action been taken which suggests that many 'cases' can be seen as organisational failures as much as personal transgression). The lists of 'charges' against the individual with their unemotive tone of objectivity attempt to nail down something of the nuanced and complex phenomenon that is poor performance. The point I am making is that the 'bad apple' explanation for nursing failures may serve certain purposes, for example 'reassuring the public' or showing the regulators' regulator that the Council has teeth but it cannot be understood as all there is to say about the matter. Nevertheless as long as it serves these functions we are likely to hear it repeated.

Finally, researcher Hannah Cooke has investigated healthcare management and disciplinary processes. One of her studies involved observation in three healthcare trusts in the north of England. She interviewed ward sisters, staff nurses, clinical nurse specialists, directorate managers and others and discussed any form of involvement in disciplinary procedures (Cooke 2006). Her findings revealed that according to her informants, punishments were commonplace but not necessarily documented. She writes 'quasi-formal discipline is often unofficial or semi-official and may happen out of the gaze of trust board managers. It is not captured in official reports on the incidence of disciplinary cases' (p. 697). Her conclusion was that quasi-official procedures were often adopted to avoid high numbers of disciplinary actions and high costs for disciplining nurses. This would also keep the actual figures of poor performance under the radar and out of the public domain. Cooke also noted that those workers that were required to attend formal disciplinary meetings, and as a result resigned or were dismissed, often went on to work in the nursing home sector. Comments were also made by her respondents regarding the apparent defensiveness of NHS culture around this topic which Cooke speculates was attached to the newly self-governing trusts who were able to discipline and suspend staff based on their own guidelines rather than national ACAS guidelines.

After that disturbing background, let me talk a little about the profile of cases that have been heard by the NMC, that is, cases that have gone further than local organisations, and their outcome.

Patterns of poor performance: Summary from NMC hearings

As I mentioned, details of most cases heard by the NMC are published on the Council's website. Recently I analysed recorded cases from the NMC records of hearings for a 6-month period (October 2009 to March 2010 inclusive). The total number of cases was 185. Records were available for the conduct and competence/professional competence committees. No details are available for health committee cases, so these were not analysed. I have summarised the results below along with an estimate of the proportion of all nurses that the number of cases represents. This can indicate if any particular types of workplace or nurses from any particular parts of the register are over-represented.

Table 6.1 shows that there are proportionately more cases involving a registered mental health nurse than for nurses on other parts of the register. Table 6.2 shows that men are significantly overrepresented.

It is not straightforward to find out whether any types of workplace are particularly associated with cases. After NHS acute trusts, the most frequent site of cases is the care home setting. However, there are a great many care homes in the United Kingdom (Table 6.3).

Professional regulators will consider disciplinary action against registrants who may have brought the profession into disrepute through problematic behaviour without a direct connection to their practice. Table 6.4 identifies that a little over one-third of cases

Table 6.1 Part of the register of nurse

	Cases	Total on register	Cases as % of all in that part
Adult registered nurse	127	396,776	0.03
Registered mental health nurse	33	61,541	0.05
Midwife (including dual registration)	15[a]	35,305	0.04
Specialist practitioner	5		
Registered child nurse	5	19,164	0.02
Learning disabilities registered nurse	2	14,187	0.01
Total	187[b]	676,547	0.03

[a]Of these, eight cases relate to midwifery practice, the rest to practice as a nurse.
[b]There is a small amount of double counting owing to registration in more than one part of the register.

Table 6.2 Gender

	Cases	Total on register	%
Male	60	72,323	0.08
Female	125	604,089	0.02
Total	185	676,412	0.03

Table 6.3 Type of NHS trust or workplace

Type of trust	Cases	% of cases	Total number in England[a]
NHS acute/hospital trust	73	39	169
Nursing or residential home	37	20	>2000
NHS mental health trust	13	7	57
NHS primary care trust	13[b]	7	152
Other independent sector	7	4	
Other	3	2	
Unknown	39	21	
Total	185	100	378

[a]Figures from Care Quality Commission for England only: http://www.cqc.org.uk/_db/_documents/CQC_Three_2009_18-4.pdf.
[b]Of these five relate to general practitioner surgeries reproduced under the Open Government Licence v1.0.

Table 6.4 Nature of case: clinically related or non-clinical, e.g. non-related criminal case

Nature of case	
Clinical	88
Clinical and non-clinical charges	18
Non-clinical	68
Unknown	11
Total	185

Table 6.5 Outcome of case

The majority of cases during the period ended in removal from the register

Outcome	
Striking off	89
Caution	49
Suspension from register	31
Conditions of practice[a] applied	16
Total	185

[a]A restriction, e.g. the nurse is forbidden to work with drugs.

concerned non-clinical charges. Clinical refers to incidents to do with patient care; non-clinical refers to other issues not directly connected to delivering patient care such as unrelated criminal convictions (Table 6.5).

Summary from NMC Fitness to Practise Annual Report 2010–2011

- During this period the NMC received 4211 potential new cases against nurses and midwives (compared with 2178 in 2008–2009) with 647 being referred to the Conduct and Competence Committee. Over 40% came from employers, 23% from members of the public, 23% from the police, and approximately 4% were anonymous.

- Of the potential 4211 new cases, it was concluded that there was no case to answer in 1847. Some 122 female and 76 male registrants were removed from the register.
- Of the incidents that the NMC hearings dealt with, 38% occurred in the NHS, and 9% came from a residential or nursing home (compared with 21% in 2008–2009), 4% came from a private hospital, and 1% involved agency nurses.
- Although the allegations concerned various issues, the most frequent complaint (25%) concerned dishonesty, for example theft. Twenty-four percent of cases concerned competency issues, 22% concerned abuse of or inappropriate relationships with patients.
- The most frequent allegations considered by the health committee were mental or physical illness (39%) and substance abuse in 27%.
- Regarding the geographical source of referrals, approximately 85% came from England, 5% from Scotland, 5% from Wales and 2% from Northern Ireland.

(Nursing and Midwifery Council 2011)

Ending off this part of the chapter, the point I want to make is that it is as well to be aware that poor performance in the NHS among nurses – and other healthcare professionals – is not always handled as well as it might be. Sometimes it is a cause for concern. However, it is important not to forget that less than 0.3% of registered nurses and midwives have their conduct investigated through fitness to practise hearings.

I now want to explore reasons for poor performance and why nurses sometimes 'fail to care'. As I hinted at the beginning, often when this topic is discussed in the media, there is an astonishing lack of insight and real knowledge about nursing on display. One often-repeated explanation is that nurses are educated at too high a level and, somehow, never develop an orientation to caring interactions with their patients. It is seen as a shame for the profession that it has 'given away' so much of the so-called basic care to healthcare support workers who are not as highly trained and, as yet, unregulated. However, as we saw in Chapter 4, such a division of labour was an almost inevitable response from healthcare managers to previous reforms in nursing education. And the most recent change in nursing education, to degree level, has been accompanied by a reduction in recruitment of trained nurses and an increase in use of support workers as managers try to cope with the latest financial pressures and cut staff costs. A more enlightened attempt to explain apparent lack of care and sometimes cruelty focuses on the emotional strain of nurses' work and a lack of support provided. Some have added the conjecture that it is specifically working with the diseased and dying that evokes strong and potentially contradictory responses from nurses, including attempts to distance themselves from their patients and a resentment that patients are 'permitted' the kind of attention that they want for themselves but feel is denied in the busy healthcare setting. It was back in 1960 that such ideas were first prominently voiced (Menzies 1960), and they have recently re-emerged (Ross 2010).

I have been talking to nurses through my research since the early 1990s, and of course spent time with nurses for much longer, and one paradoxical and puzzling thing has struck me that is so much part of the air of nursing that it is easy to no longer notice it. This is that nurses often express highly negative talk about nursing work with a high degree of energy and even a kind of enjoyment. Particular phrases are repeated, in focus groups or interviews I, or colleagues, have held over time and across continents. Even with a short acquaintance with nursing and midwifery, you may have noticed the same. Ideas from psychoanalysis can suggest some explanations for this strange observation. Psychoanalysis points out that all of us, not just nurses, behave in contradictory ways, as we attempt to avoid facing up to certain realities and to persist in our fantasies. Psychoanalytic theory offers explanations that include the possibility that our motivations for talking and acting might be largely unknown to us. The father of psychoanalysis, Sigmund Freud (1856–1939), developed the notion of the unconscious that influences how we experience and act in the world without our knowledge or assent, sometimes in counter-intuitive ways. He subjected his theory to rigorous scientific investigation by means of analytic conversations with his patients. He claimed that the influence of the unconscious was observable in dreams, slips of the tongue and in jokes. Apart from having an origin in clinical work, psychoanalytic theory has been used in the interpretation of various cultural phenomena such as organisational or even national behaviour.[3] So why might nurses appear to enjoy extreme negativity about their work so much, and why do they sometimes lose a sense of standards to such an extent that patients suffer?

Let me first set out the skeleton of my four-part argument before I go on to flesh it out:

- Nursing promotes an idealised vision of nursing work and of the identity of the nurse as fully caring and fully autonomous. Such roles are, according to some psychoanalytic theory, inherently 'blocked' and impossible.
- Faced with an everyday experience that is strongly at odds with this vision, nurses look for an explanation of this fact that is based on external constraints. They do this because this provokes less anxiety than fundamentally questioning a prevailing ideology in nursing.
- In addition to this, there is a particular kind of pleasure found by nurses in repeating accounts of their apparently powerless position. Feeling one's self to be a victim can provide a sense of having 'moral high ground'.
- This pleasure in powerlessness, and willingness to be 'flexible' or do your duty no matter the cost is a feature of nursing that is essential for its functioning within the structures of healthcare systems but brings about a kind of acquiescence that makes nurses less likely to challenge poor practice.

In Chapter 1, I discussed the way that nursing has been presented by the profession – in moral and religious terms initially which gave way, during the mid-20th century, to a humanistic emphasis, calling

---

[3] For the application of psychoanalytic theory to politics and culture, see the writing of Slovenian Marxist psychoanalyst Slavoj Žižek, for example Žižek, S. (2005). *Interrogating the Real*. London, Continuum.

nurses into no less a grand project. Professional autonomy, status and respect have been constant themes. We could call these representations idealistic, ideological or fictions. In addition to this kind of impossibility, some psychoanalysts claim that any role or any identity is impossible or blocked for the simple reason that the human subject is, according to them, a divided subject (divided into ego and unconscious for example). So how might nursing and individual nurses respond in the face of this injunction embedded in nursing discourse to be fulfilled, autonomous professionals? At an institutional level there might be a willingness to confuse what actually happens with the ideal, that is, to idealise – 'we are already autonomous' – or we might see convoluted definitions of autonomy – 'we are fully autonomous within our own sphere of activity'. These idealisations are all available to individual nurses; however unsanctioned talk of negativity, indignation and victimhood, which would be out of place on the podium or in the board room, offers paradoxical opportunities for satisfaction.

Look at an extract taken from research that I was involved in during the early 1990s. This was a national project examining job satisfaction among British nurses after major changes to the NHS. The study involved the collection of written comments from nurses and also included my field notes from staff meetings that I attended across England. Both data sources featured a great many descriptions of self-sacrifice and expressions of indignation and powerlessness, as below:

> *Health visitor*: 'The care that patients/clients get is due to the commitment of the individual nurses including myself. I like to do my job to the best of my ability and put myself out in order to do it i.e. come in early, do without lunch, etc'.
> *Clinical Nurse Specialist*: I do a lot of overtime in order to finish my work and give the patients the care they are entitled to have, but of course do not get paid for this.
> Field notes November, 1992 P. Community Health Services: An HV (health visitor) told the group, 'No one has personally said [this] but an ethos is dripping down and the ethos is money. It's

> always money'. 'Is there anything that you can do, faced with all this?' I asked. The reply was: 'We're pretty much pawns in some of this. You can't fight against the power of money'.

A colleague[4] conducted research into nurse retention in Melbourne, Australia, in 2010. The last extract is from her focus group data:

> *Nurse 1:* ...they'll [doctors] allow you to do so much when the mood suits them, like they're going out for the night, but when the mood doesn't suit them they're very quick to put you in your place.
>
> *Nurse 2:* ...for the junior staff, it stops them from speaking up again, you know.... They'll think twice before they think to voice an opinion unless they've got a charge nurse who'll be their advocate...not only are the patients your clients but the doctors are also your clients. So who are the nurses?
> [muffled word and laughter from the other nurses] What did you say?
>
> *Nurse 1:* The slaves!...

These are just two short extracts, but they represent a much larger body of similar talk where nurses present themselves as exploited by a powerful other, and appear to derive a kind of energy from talking about this. One group even describe themselves, humorously, as 'the slaves'. I'd like to suggest that there are two reasons for this kind of talk being so widespread. Unspoken in these particular quotations is the assumption that these nurses, and perhaps nursing as a whole, would be able to achieve the full potential set out by the ideal/ideological versions of the profession discussed earlier if

---

[4] Alicia Evans from the Australian Catholic University, Melbourne. Alicia is a Lacanian psychoanalyst.

only nurses were not prevented by outside forces – usually the out-side forces are doctors but more recently they include managers and patients and their relatives, or staff shortages or bureaucracy. It is less challenging to keep the fantasy intact than to face the pos-sibility that the basis for how I think about myself and the work I do is ultimately a fiction. The second reason is that identification with victimhood offers a number of benefits. If nurses can impute guilt to others, they can present themselves as innocent, and gain deep satisfaction of founding their identity on a collective injury (Žižek 2005). It absolves them from taking responsibility, perhaps even from resisting organisational interventions that lead to poor standards of care.

But, you might ask, don't workers in many occupations complain about their conditions? Isn't it always easier to complain than to take action? What makes nurses so unusual? What makes nurses unusual, I think, is the vestige of the moral and religious orienta-tion to duty and even self-sacrifice that lingers in the profession as a whole. This makes the kind of talk I've quoted here familiar and acceptable. Perhaps it subtly influences individuals to stay 'at the bedside' when the conditions of work have become unbearable and destructive. I would even go as far as to suggest that many health systems rely on this general passivity within their large nursing work-force for their functioning. The official talk in the United Kingdom is that the NHS needs nurses who can innovate, challenge, take responsibility, manage, etc., but the overriding experience is that nurses are expected to make the NHS work from day to day, manag-ing an increasing throughput and dependency, sometimes with little organisational authority along with maximum exposure to patient suffering.

Inquiries: What went wrong?

Before leaving the topic of serious failures in health care, I want to present and discuss the results of inquiries into a few of the more notorious cases. These are the inquiry into peripartum hysterectomy at Our Lady of Lourdes Hospital, Drogheda, Ireland, published in

2006, the report of the public inquiry into children's heart surgery in Bristol published in 2001 and the final report of the independent inquiry into care provided by Mid Staffordshire NHS Foundation Trust, England, which was published in 2010. The full report of this last failure, the Francis Report, is due to be released as I write. I want to do this because the authors of reports or chairs of inquiry panels all make it clear that when cultures develop that allow poor standards of health care to continue unchallenged, there is a failure across all the groups involved in care delivery and management, not just nurses. The argument I am making in this part of the chapter points to what I consider unique features of nursing that can account for its part in failures, but I am not for a moment suggesting that nurses are any more culpable than other groups. In fact it is often nurses who do blow the whistle on poor practice and in the process 'open Pandora's box'.

The Inquiry into peripartum hysterectomy at Our Lady of Lourdes Hospital, Drogheda, its report published in 2006, was instigated to examine the reasons for an unacceptably high rate of hysterectomies over a period of many years for young women, carried out particularly by one obstetrician who worked there. Hysterectomy carried out at the time of a caesarean section is a remedy of last resort for uncontrollable and life-threatening blood loss, but the rates of this particular procedure were unusually high in this hospital. The doctor in question was suspended and eventually struck off; however, one of the key questions that the inquiry posed was why this bad practice had been allowed to continue for so long – for many decades. A number of midwives had voiced concerns but no action had been taken. The judge who carried out the inquiry wrote

> We tried to understand why the midwives, who formed the largest group of health professionals involved and who were principled women of training and intelligence, did not take their concerns further. Why did they not speak to management? Why did they not bring their concerns to the Matron and her assistant? ... The sad reality was that the Matron of the Maternity Unit was not given the power to properly administer the Maternity Unit. She

lacked the authority necessary to question the consultants or to change procedures, and she lacked the support of the [owners of the hospital] if a dispute arose ... Her long years working with the [hospital owners] moulded her into a caring and deeply committed, but submissive nurse with no confidence to take her concerns to a higher level, or to follow through on them. Many of the nurses we interviewed fitted the same mould.

(Harding Clark, M 2006: 156–186)

My second example, the 'Bristol Inquiry', was a landmark event for medicine and for the NHS in the United Kingdom. The Bristol Royal Infirmary and the Bristol Royal Hospital for Sick Children were teaching hospitals associated with Bristol University's Medical School and looked after patients with heart disease: adults, children and infants. From the late 1980s, concerns were expressed about the mortality rate for particular surgical procedures for babies with congenital heart disease. The concerns turned into complaints to the GMC, and two surgeons were struck off and a further disciplined. A public inquiry was opened in 1998. Its remit was partly to conduct a factual inquiry into events and partly to make proposals for improvements in care. The report of the inquiry is, unsurprisingly, long and detailed and concluded that the problem was 'multifactoral and multidisciplinary' (Kennedy, Bristol Royal Infirmary Inquiry et al. 2001: 23). Much of it details the moving evidence from parents of babies treated there and from doctors. The report's authors have this to say about nurses in general and a small number of nurses in particular:

We regard it as significant that we did not hear concerns being brought to senior figures at the UBH/T [United Bristol Healthcare NHS Trust] by the nursing staff. We do not infer from this any lack of concern on the part of nurses. Rather, we see it as illustrating a larger truth. The hierarchical system common at the time (and regrettably still too prevalent now) made it difficult for the nursing staff to voice concerns and to be heard. It is revealing that only when independent experts from outside the UBHT

[...] came to carry out their review, did Fiona Thomas feel able to express her concerns about the lack of proper organisation in the ICU. It is also indicative of the state of affairs that the only way which Kay Armstrong and Mona Herborn felt was open to them to make known their dissatisfaction with aspects of PCS [pae-diatric cardiac surgery] was to withdraw their services from the operating theatre when a switch operation was to be performed. Nursing staff were let down by a culture that excluded them.

(Kennedy, Bristol Royal Infirmary Inquiry et al. 2001: 175)

The third and most recent of the 'scandals' focussed on the Mid Staffordshire NHS Foundation Trust in England. Concerns about mortality and the standard of care provided in this trust resulted in an investigation by the Healthcare Commission (now the Care Quality Commission) which published a highly critical report in March 2009. This was followed by two reviews commissioned by the Department of Health. These investigations gave rise to widespread public concern and a loss of confidence in the trust (Francis 2010: 7). At the time of writing, a public inquiry is drawing to a close but the independent inquiry chaired by Robert Francis QC provides a great deal of detail about the kind of incidents that occurred partic-ularly in Stafford Hospital, and often featuring nursing care. Unlike the previous reports I have presented, this did not come to any over-all conclusion about nursing culture as such but did comment that nurses were fearful of giving evidence to the inquiry and that:

the nursing staff in particular, are thoroughly demoralised as a result of the events of the last few years. I believe that many have adopted a survival strategy of going through the motions of doing their job as opposed to pursuing a much valued and necessary vocation. (p. 412)

The report identified a number of contributing factors to the trust's poor performance. One that has gained some prominence is that the trust's management became too focussed on meeting targets and reducing costs. Partly as a result of this staffing levels were inadequate. One accident and emergency doctor said this to the inquiry:

> The problem was primarily that there just were not enough staff... Nobody comes to work, very few people come to work to do a bad job, and I have never met a nurse who comes to work to do a bad job. The nurses were so under-resourced that they were working extra hours, they were desperately moving from place to place to try to give adequate care to patients. If you are in that environment for long enough, what happens is you become immune to the sound of pain. You either become immune to the sound of pain or you walk away. You cannot feel people's pain, you cannot continue to want to do the best you possibly can when the system says no to you, you can't do the best you can. And the system in the hospital said no to the nursing staff doing the best they could and to the doctors, but I think the nursing staff probably feel that more acutely in certain respects. (p. 190)

At the time of writing, a popular UK media style of reality documentary features the secretly filmed abuse of vulnerable patients by nurses or other paid carers in hospitals and care homes (BBC Panorama 2011). These come in the wake of a series of government inquiries and reports which identify failures of fundamental health care, concerning dignity and nutrition for older people (CQC 2011), sometimes with events leading to deaths (BBC News 2010) and often with nurses heavily implicated (Health Service Ombudsman 2011). The metamorphosis of care into cruelty gives rise to public expressions of shock and incomprehension and responses from professional bodies of outrage along with assurances that the majority of health care delivered is satisfactory (NMC 2011; RCN 2011).

I want to suggest that this mystery of poor care (where it involves nurses – and not all of these scandals do) is the price paid for the supreme flexibility that a generally unempowered workforce provides the health service. Those working as nurses are likely to experience a unique combination of tensions. Healthcare systems require their employees to deal with highly stressful and potentially traumatic events, perhaps on a daily basis. In addition, these organisations feature a division of labour and of responsibility and differences in levels of training of their professional groups that result in nurses working in close proximity to trauma but, certainly in the case of the organisations that formed the subject of the inquiries I have discussed, lacking the organisational authority or the knowledge to act and make decisions, a situation described in work psychological literature as 'high demand low control' (Karasek, Brisson et al. 1998).

I end this potentially depressing chapter by repeating what I wrote in the introduction to this book – that you don't address a problem by ignoring or minimising it. When things go wrong in health care, the reasons are usually extremely complicated, and although it's fair to say that each practitioner is responsible for what they do, the context they practice in can make it relatively easy or difficult to act in accordance with the highest standards. I am not convinced that requiring nurses to complete a year of hands-on caring before training, as the final Francis report recommends, will address the problems highlighted in this chapter.

7

Health Policy and Politics: Targets, Managerialism and Funding

If you work as a nurse or doctor – or a dentist or any other of the clinical trades – and you work for the National Health Service (NHS), you work in a highly politicised setting. Paradoxically, even when governments are 'giving clinicians autonomy', it can feel like interference. The NHS has presented a major vulnerability for centre-left governments, as it remains one of the pillars of welfare in the United Kingdom, upon which values of collectivism are judged. For more right-wing governments, it has represented some of the worst aspects of state-funded monopolies rife with waste, bureaucracy and lack of concern for its users. This chapter sets out why and how the UK NHS has been so highly politicised and what this means for practising nurses. It asks whether the NHS has got better since major reforms of the 1980s and 1990s. It focuses on how recent governments have understood the place of nursing, often seeing it as a more pliable group than doctors, open to more influence and able to be used as a policy instrument. The appearance (and disappearance) of 'modern matrons', 'nurse consultants' and 'nurse entrepreneurs' are discussed.

It's Tuesday 27 April 2010. The RCN's annual congress in Bournemouth is in full swing. There's an unusual energy this year. A double-decked bus is parked just outside the venue. It is bathed in TV lighting, and so many press photographers are crowding around it that it is hard to get back into the Bournemouth International Centre where congress is being held. Its Nick Clegg's Vote Lib Dem campaign bus and apparently the bus has been touring the country, attracting similar attention in an attempt to encourage people, unsurprisingly, to vote Lib Dem.[1] The following Thursday is polling day in the United Kingdom's general election, and as one of the largest public sector unions, the RCN's high profile congress is not to be missed by politicians of any party. Gordon Brown, then Labour prime minister, in almost his last week of office was there on Monday, telling the audience that he wants to see more nurse specialists and greater autonomy for nurses, and that while NHS management costs will be reduced by one-third, front line care will be protected. Nick Clegg, leader of the Liberal Democrats, is there the day after Gordon, wearing a yellow tie. He promises his party would preserve NHS spending, 'If the axe falls on caring staff', he says, 'it will cost us all more in the long term'. Finally Andrew Lansley, soon to be health secretary in the new Conservative-Liberal coalition, addresses congress for just under 50 minutes. His main theme is that NHS staff know best how to run the service, and that he will make sure that the NHS has autonomy to ensure there is 'no political interference day by day'. He also wants to see 'new opportunities for leadership for nurses' and claims that the NHS budget would be 'protected and increasing'. His closing remark, in reply to a question from the floor about why nurses should vote Conservative, is 'A lot of it's about policy, but to me ... it's actually fundamentally about people'. In this chapter I ask 'which people'?

What is policy?

Let's say policy is something like 'a formal course of action proposed or adopted'. Any group of people can make a policy. A clothes shop will have a returns policy for its goods, a family with young children a television-watching policy or a hospital a hand-washing

---

[1] The double-decker bus has a particular, and positive, place in the British imagination. Not only has it become a symbol of London, and by extension things British, but a double-decker bus played the main role in Cliff Richard's 1963 classic film *Summer Holiday*.

policy. So policy would involve courses of action to bring something about or formalised responses to particular situations. The policies made by one group of people may affect another group who had no part in the policy-making process. Policies may protect the interests of the group from which policy makers emerge, as in the case of the clothes returns policy. Usually policies have explicit desired outcomes, though sometimes they have unintended and unwanted consequences. The more complex is the context in which the policy operates, the more likely are unintended consequences. Sometimes unintended consequences are a result of different groups having different interests. The notion of 'perverse' effects describes when a policy sets up incentives for a particular group that bring about the very opposite effect that the policy intended. For example, it is in the interests of the clothes shop to receive as few returned dresses as possible but it is in customers' interests to be able to return dresses when they wish. The clothes shop develops a policy where it will only accept returned clothes which are faulty. Customers realise that the only way they can return dresses they realise don't fit or they don't want is to damage them in some way. The shop therefore ends up with a large amount of returned and damaged merchandise which it cannot resell.

Though some principles are similar, government policy is of a different order of scale and complexity to these examples. First is the complex notion of the democratic mandate of governments. There is an assumption that a political party that receives the most votes in an election has won the right to put the policies it devises into action (see the next chapter for views about mandate and democracy from leading nurses). However, political parties regularly devise policies and actions that appear to be supported by very few members of the public, such as the decision to invade Iraq in 2003 which has widely been associated with the beliefs of a single individual, the then prime minister, Tony Blair. Some policies appear to further the interests of certain groups who are perhaps seen as key supporters of particular parties. An example might be employment policy that makes it easier for employers to sack workers. The second difference of scale is that political parties have, or present themselves as having (or sometimes deny having), an organised set of beliefs and values about what society is and should be, the nature of the barriers to these goals and how these should be addressed. We might call this ideology.

> **What is ideology?** Ideology has been understood and defined sometimes in ways that emphasise that it is something illusory, distorted or mystifying and sometimes as sets of ideas that organise social, cultural and economic life. The second use does not foreground the issue of truth or falsehood but rather emphasises the impossibility that any cultural practice does not emerge from some set of presuppositions. Ideology does not have to be explicit or conscious to be effective. In fact it is most effective when it is not.

Sometimes these can involve fundamental beliefs about human characteristics and motivation, for example about whether individuals are largely motivated by self-interest or by maintaining solidarity with others. These often form part, or the main part of their policies. In fact the use of policy to achieve social ends is relatively recent. In the late 19th century many states had taken up responsibility for 'public goods' such as sanitation and public health, but it was after the Second World War and then during the 1960s that they used social policy more actively to combat problems such as poverty or ill-health.

How is policy made? By which people?

I now want to return to the question posed earlier. Andrew Lansley claimed that as a policy maker, he remained focussed on the person who would be affected by his policies. I want to ask who are the people who shape policy? Many forces and groups influence the formation and implementation of policy, and an examination of how this occurs has been a major strand in the study of government. The short answer is that it is a complex mix of government ideology, policy communities including pressure groups, popular media pressures and perceived public acceptability.

Ideology – I have referred to ideology earlier. While it is unavoidable that ideology drives policy, because a belief about what would be a preferred state of affairs is inevitably ideological, it no longer seems believable that the United Kingdom's major political parties offer contrasting ideologies. This will become clear when I describe New Labour's health policy from 1997 onwards which earned comments that it dared go further than Margaret Thatcher in terms of introducing 'market forces' into health care, for example.

Pressure groups – While the role of political parties in a democracy is to seek to attain power, the aim of pressure groups is to influence power, or, more particularly, the making of public policy (Kavanagh 2006). We can classify pressure groups in a number of ways. The first set is promotional, cause or attitude-based groups which would include those campaigning for reform to abortion law, for example, and the 'think-tanks' representing views across the political spectrum. A second group would be sectional or interest groups. These would include occupational groups, trade unions and business groups such as those representing pharmaceutical or tobacco interests. The most useful distinction, however, if we are trying to account for which groups have influence, is that between insider and outsider groups. Insider groups are those which have regular contact with policy makers in the relevant government department. They tend to have information and expertise the government needs and speak with authority for their sector. And though their aims would be broadly aligned to government policy, they also have the power to veto policy, in theory at least. The Thatcher government, however, set on public sector reform, took a confrontational approach toward groups that represented public sector providers. For that government, these groups were part of the national problem of self-interest and resistance to change that it sought to defeat. Perhaps since then governments of the 'right' and 'left' have expected resistance and disagreement from these groups toward their reforms. The most recent reorganisation of the NHS, introduced by Andrew Lansley during 2011 and 2012, seems to have encountered an unprecedented amount of opposition from the main medical and nursing organisations, resulting in them being excluded from key consultation meetings.

Media pressures – The operation of, and usually, apparent failure of the health service makes good (in the sense of successful) news stories, both in local and national press. Governments have taken enormous pains to win the support of the popular media, as recent revelations about the close relationship between senior government figures and powerful news executives have shown in the United Kingdom (see http://www.levesoninquiry.org.uk/). It is not far-fetched therefore to include the avoidance of unwelcome media attention as a driver of health policy. Stories of long-waiting times (particularly in emergency departments), then of dirty hospital wards and hospital-acquired infections, were followed by directives aimed at solving these problems from the Department of Health during the years of the New Labour administration. The relationship between 'public opinion' and the media is complex, but the two are related and politicians note that communications to them from constituents tend to 'follow the headlines'.

A brief summary of health policy in the United Kingdom

A number of books exist discussing social policy, and many of these are written specifically for nurses. Because of this I only give the briefest outline of UK health – or rather healthcare – policy here.

The National Health Service was set up in 1948 after the end of the Second World War as part of a wave of welfarism and humanism that swept Europe and North America in response to the horrors of war.[2] Its principle is broadly one of shared risk. The service is largely funded from taxation, and for the most part its services are free to those judged to need them. However, any insurance-based system of health care needs to solve several major problems (Strong and Robinson 1990): health is a fundamental human prerequisite, yet health and disease are so complex that most of the population have no choice but to rely on the judgements of those experts whom they engage to address their health needs. This creates the possibility of 'supplier-induced demand', i.e. that doctors or

---

[2] It is the German Chancellor Otto von Bismark, however, who is credited with setting up the first social insurance-based health and welfare system in the 1880s. He wore a hat with a spike on top. Check for yourself.

others might 'over-supply' their paid services. The second dilemma concerns the financial viability of the whole system, partly because those most in need of the service may well be the least able to pay, and partly because with technological and pharmaceutical development, healthcare costs are likely to be continually rising. The NHS attempted to overcome the first problem by paying doctors not for each item of service but a salary. In addition it set up a system of general practitioners (GPs) who act as the gatekeepers to consultant care for the population. The second problem was addressed by the sheer scope and size of a national service in which the whole population was enrolled. Although a substantial success, the NHS had some built-in problems. According to many commentators, chief among these was the enormous power of the medical profession.[3] The deals done to ensure medical support for the establishment of the service gave doctors, and perhaps especially hospital doctors, some highly attractive working conditions, notably huge freedom (Strong and Robinson 1990: 15.)

In addition, because of the complexity and fundamental nature of medical work, no outsider possessed the competence to dare to judge the work of a doctor. If doctors were also empowered to make decisions about resources (to buy expensive new equipment for example), then this could make central financial control all but impossible. Two other linked problems also existed: the frugality of the service led to sometimes lengthy waiting lists for treatment, and it was virtually impossible to change GP or to choose your hospital consultant. In other words, patients were subordinate to those who provided care.

No end to the changes

Most readers of this book will know that the NHS has undergone an apparently relentless series of reorganisations. The driving force

---

[3] Historian of nursing Susan McGann tells how the civil servants working on the creation of the National Health Service felt that they did not have to consult with nursing's leaders, simply because as women, in the 1940s, they could be ignored.

behind nearly all of them has been to address these problems left behind in the original design of the system.

The drama of many of the earlier changes has now settled into the sediment of the health service over the decades, but the effects linger. I want to single out one strand before turning to look at how nursing and nurses have fared in healthcare policy. That policy strand has worked, over the last 30 years, to increase central control over the NHS by means of strengthened management. A number of forces came together to bring this about. The 1980s saw a series of powerfully influential books by corporate managers, and management consultants,[4] who talked up the potential role of leadership in organisations; at the same time critiques of professionalism, including of medical dominance were gaining visibility (see Chapters 3 and 4). Governments began to look to the private sector for inspiration for ways to increase the efficiency of the NHS, and the first big idea to be tried was general management, that is that powerful managers could set objectives for their organisation, analyse and if necessary change structures and processes, and monitor and measure performance. The idea that what was needed was *management* skill rather than expertise in any particular area was a direct challenge to professional medical power. Instead of an unorganised set of plans and solutions negotiated privately by a hospital's consultants, each possibly competing with each other for resources and power, it could be that one person take overall responsibility for the direction of and work done within a healthcare organisation. This vision was hugely attractive to governments faced with spiralling healthcare costs. Some doctors and nurses were lured into these roles, but they were often reviled by their professional peers.

An even more audacious idea (on the part of Margaret Thatcher's Conservative government) emerged in the early 1990s. It involved the splitting of the whole service in two, into those parts which made decisions about the scale and type of services needed by populations

---

[4] For example Peters and Waterman's In Search of Excellence. Peters, T. and R. Waterman (1982). *In Search of Excellence*. New York, Harper and Row.

and those which 'provided' them. The idea was that 'commissioners' including GPs could shop around for the most efficient and responsive services for their populations or patients. This was intended to incentivise organisations to consider both costs and the quality of their services as, in theory, the 'customers' could go elsewhere. In practice this barely happened, and the whole purchaser–provider structure was dismantled by the Labour government when it came to power in 1997.

> By the end of the Conservative rule, the UK NHS was among the least well funded in Europe. In 1986 the health and social care budget amounted to 5.7% of the UK gross domestic product. In 2008–2009, after a dozen years of Labour administration, the proportion of its allocation rose to 9.5%.

Scrutiny and control under New Labour

New Labour's arrival in 1997 was marked by pledges to abolish the internal market. Apart from its ideological unacceptability, the internal market was seen to lead to some sharp inequalities in local service provision. Health policy is always at least in part driven by high profile media concerns, and New Labour's promise to spend the savings from scrapping the internal market on reducing waiting lists and waiting times was no exception and marks the continuing prominence of this long-standing problem. The early days of New Labour were peppered by press reports of patients left for hours or even days on trolleys waiting for hospital beds to become available. By December of their first year in office, it had started to establish national standards of treatment and a programme of NHS 'modernisation'. The founding of a Commission for Health Improvement (CHI), and National Institute of Clinical Excellence (NICE) in 1999, marks a key moment in New Labour Health policy. For the first time since the conception of the NHS, a central body scientifically investigated the medical benefit and assessed the cost-effectiveness of different treatments and issued guidelines to the service, sometimes, not unpredictably, causing controversy. CHI, later subsumed into the Healthcare Commission, was the first body ever to assess the clinical performance of NHS providers and report the results publicly, also carrying out investigations where serious failures were apparent (see Chapter 6). Performance was now, at least beginning to be, open to central scrutiny and control in a way never before attempted in the UK NHS. As I have mentioned in previous chapters, medical scandals such as the failure of children's heart surgery at the Bristol Royal Infirmary between 1984 and 1995 and the multiple murders of his patients by GP Harold Shipman during the 1990s created a context where control over medical activity was seen as an overdue priority for any government. Performance indicators were set out, and in September 2001 the government published the first performance ratings for NHS trusts providing acute hospital services. This was followed in subsequent years by ratings for other sectors of the service as well as the setting out and enforcement of various targets for performance, notably to do with waiting times.[5]

The micro-management of NHS performance became one of the more controversial features of the Blair government. With an increasing range of performance and quality data being collected by the Department of Health, and the abolition of intermediary NHS Regional Authorities, the way was open for 'career-limiting' telephone calls direct from the Secretary of State to Chief Executives of struggling NHS trusts. If the measurement of performance was conducted with scientific principles, the same cannot be said about the government's approach to performance management. During their time in office, New Labour achieved a level of command and control that their predecessors only dreamed of.

Labour also attempted to modernise the hearts and minds of NHS personnel. A number of, often short-lived, agencies such as the Modernisation Agency, formed in 2003 and replaced 2 years later by the

---

[5] An extremely useful and highly readable account of policy under New Labour is available at the NHS History website, currently at http://www.nhshistory.net/chapter_6.html.

NHS Institute for Improvement and Innovation, were created aiming to promote innovative thinking and break entrenched ways of working. A key part of its 'modernising' aim was to mount a challenge to traditional professional demarcations.

New Labour policy priorities can be seen in terms of two phases: from 2003 to 2006 improving access and reducing waiting, and from 2004 to 2008 increasing patient choice and the range of healthcare providers. This is a second area where the Blair government outdid the Thatcher regime. The thinking was that if the independent or private sector could provide a service in a more timely, acceptable or efficient way, then the NHS could purchase such services for the benefit of its patients. The government passed legislation enabling and in some cases even requiring commissioners to contract with a range of service providers.

In the last analysis, the Blair reforms and the major investment made by his government produced mixed results. Although performance in the service improved on many measures, and more information was made available in the public domain, the salaries of healthcare personnel improved and waiting times reduced, other problems either remained or emerged. Health inequalities did not respond to various initiatives though the fact that the United Kingdom has seen three Commissions on the topic in the last 40 years, and a number of initiatives, shows its importance to policy makers of both major parties. Second, shocking failures of service or failures to respect patient dignity have come into view, and it is hard not to connect these to some extent with a culture where NHS organisations and their leaders are placed under great pressure to meet certain targets, targets that sometimes look as if they are derived more from the desire to avoid media embarrassment than from coordinated system-wide priorities. I discussed this in Chapter 6.

Nurses and UK health policy

Some have argued that governments have focussed such attention on attempts to bring medicine under its control, that the much larger but less troublesome nursing profession has been caught in policy largely in an indirect way (Robinson 1997). Perhaps it was New Labour, more than any other administration, that has used nursing to achieve its policy objectives. These concerned streamlining and making NHS patient processes more efficient partly by reducing professional demarcation, increasing the choice of services available to patients, making up the reduction in hours worked by junior doctors,[6] dealing with recruitment problems in nursing and enabling the more 'flexible' nursing profession to encroach on territory previously held by medicine. Tony Blair's various secretaries of state for health introduced a series of innovations presented as beneficial for nursing but which, according to rumour at the time, sometimes came as a surprise to nursing's leaders.

The *Nurse-led NHS Direct* – This was announced in *The New NHS Modern Dependable* (Department of Health 1997). This telephone service was hoped to considerably reduce GP and emergency department work and opened up a new career opportunity for nurses.

Nurse consultants, along with Midwife and Health Visitor Consultants, were first proposed in the Department of Health strategy document *Making a Difference* published in 1999 (Department of Health 1999). This document emphasised that 'nurses and nursing were valued, and should be more powerful'. It proposed that these new nursing roles could provide a stronger focus for clinical leadership and expanded, 'modernised', roles for nurses. It also announced further extension to nurse prescribing which had been first introduced in 1994.

Modern matrons – *The NHS Plan* (Department of Health 2000) promoted a new clinical nursing leader the 'modern matrons who, it claimed, would be given authority to troubleshoot basic ward-level problems that had dominated in the media such as lack of cleanliness and hospital-acquired infection.

In April 2001 Alan Milburn, the Secretary of State, said that matrons would be brought back but the new role was not that of

---

[6] The European Working Time Directive (EWTD) came into effect for doctors in training in August 2004.

past matrons ... Their job was to be visible, with the authority to get things done, lead the nursing team in groups of wards, demonstrate to other nurses the high standards NHS patients should expect, make sure patients got quality care, and that cleaning and food standards were met ... They might be concerned with infection control, and might have the power to order tests, admit and discharge patients, run clinics, triage patients and, where appropriate, prescribe medicines ... Over the next few years increasing numbers were appointed. The numbers in the grade of 'nurse consultant' or 'modern matron' grew to over 1000 in 2007.

Rivett (2011)

'Ten key roles' for nurses announced by the Chief Nursing Officer in England, many of which were previously undertaken by doctors (see Chapter 4 for detail).

Expanded roles for nurses and promotion of *'Nurse entrepreneurs'* and nurse partners in GP practices promoted by John Reid in 2003:

Nurse prescribing sends a powerful message to the public and others that nursing is not subservient to medicine but an equal part of the healthcare team .... – let's have more nurses employing more doctors.

Department of Health (2003)

Although there was enthusiasm for these new posts, many employers created roles hastily with the result that the work carried out, by modern matrons for example, varied widely (Savage and Scott 2004), and many in post felt that they did not have the organisational authority that the government rhetoric promised (Koteyko and Nerlich 2008). It has been claimed that nurses are often excluded from high-level policy making (Robinson and Elkan 1992), and we can see the policy attention outlined above as driven, not by the profession, but by changing NHS political pressures and priorities (see my interview with the Chief Nursing Officer in the next chapter to support this claim). Reflecting a concern with NHS efficiency, the Chief Nursing Officer's new 10 roles for nurses, included in the NHS Plan, featured new organisational and administrative roles alongside clinical roles e.g. ordering tests, managing caseloads, prescribing drugs. In 2000 and 2001 when patient waiting lists and their manipulation by some trusts were a high profile political problem (Carvel and Allison 2001), *The NHS Plan CNO's message to nurses* (March 2001) emphasised that new nursing roles could improve patients' journeys through the healthcare system. Nurses could reduce waiting and aid access to the system by providing additional points of access. Nursing role substitution for doctors was also promoted as a mechanism for addressing another key government objective, that of increasing patient choice. Alongside other mechanisms for encouraging diversity of provider which were introduced particularly in primary care (Crisp 2005), new nursing roles in walk-in centres, GP surgeries, nurse-led clinics in various specialities and the telephone service NHS Direct were presented as nurses' specific contribution to this major objective and as alternatives to making an appointment to see a GP.

The most recent NHS changes

This chapter would not be complete without giving an outline of the latest reorganisation of the NHS, currently in the process of implementation. Although there have been a great many reorganisations of the service, this particular plan met with such strong opposition from professional organisations, health unions and within the House of Commons and of Lords that the passing of the Bill was delayed for a 'listening exercise' after which some 1,000 changes were made in a (largely unsuccessful) attempt to appease critics. The Bill was given royal assent more than a year after it was first presented to the House of Commons. The British Medical Association, the Royal College of Nursing and the Royal College of Midwives expressed complete opposition to the Bill.

Under the plans, GPs and other clinicians were given much more responsibility for spending the NHS budget in England, while greater competition with the private sector was to be encouraged. The 10 strategic health authorities and 151 primary care trusts which planned and commissioned services were abolished and replaced with a national Board, two further tiers and 240 commissioning groups. In the initial plans commissioning was to be undertaken by GPs on behalf of their communities, but after questions about their readiness, and willingness, for such an important role, other clinicians, including nurses, were included in these groups. The reforms were also designed to encourage more participation and competition from the private health sector, and this has proved one of the greatest areas of controversy. The involvement of the private and voluntary sectors were enabled and encouraged under New Labour, but in practice the level of involvement was low. The latest reforms are considered to allow a greater degree of private involvement. This, along with anticipated considerable savings from reducing management roles,[7] is said to be necessary by the government in the face of potentially escalating healthcare costs due to a rising burden of diseases such as obesity and an ageing population. The changes came into effect in April 2013.

Apart from concerns over 'privatisation of the NHS' (NHS hospitals would be allowed to do 49% of their work in the private sector), many critics believe that it is foolhardy to undertake such a major restructuring at the same time that the service is being required to make £20bn of savings by 2015 as part of public sector cuts. Many commentators believe that the case for the need for change has not convincingly been made to NHS staff.

It is of course too early to say what the effect has been. Generally the impacts of such changes are complex with benefits in some areas and some unanticipated (or by some completely predictable and anticipated) problems. Often implementation is uneven or poorly carried out, and a new range of changes are launched while the first change is still having an effect so it becomes impossible to carry out any objective and rigorous evaluation. Promoters of the change (there seem few in this case) will produce examples and statistics to support the initiative, and critics will bring out counter-examples. It seems likely that the significant reduction in overall NHS budget,

---

[7] The government claimed that the reduction in staff would save £5bn by 2015.

which according to the RCN is reducing nursing posts, and not only the management layers as was claimed by Andrew Lansley, will have the largest effect on the NHS and the quality of the service it provides over the next 2–3 years.

Public health

In this chapter the focus has been on policy for healthcare organisation and delivery. Health policy more broadly includes attention to public health issues, and a great many advocates of the need for governments to have a broader view of health have pointed out that preventive, public health interventions have potentially far more impact than increased spending on curative services. These would include initiatives designed to discourage such public ills as obesity, inactivity, smoking, drug and alcohol misuse and accidents. It includes sexual health and maternal and child health and also initiatives outside of the health sector that promote and enable positive health such as those to do with housing or transport.

The UK NHS remains an enigma: high degrees of personal dedication from its staff but poor morale, national campaigns for patient dignity but shameful system failures, powerful medical elites who feel disempowered by managers, massive investment (in the past) but insolvent hospitals, loved by the public but scandals rarely out of the news. As I showed from speeches by politicians to the RCN in 2010, in the approach to the UK general election, none of the major political parties dared speak of outright cuts to services, though the supposedly proliferating number of managers and the need for 'increased efficiency' were repeated. The most recent changes to the NHS met with fierce resistance from medical and nursing organisations. Nevertheless, the careful phrases that politicians from all parties had been using give an indication that the status of the service as quasi-religion for the British public is something that no one dares unsettle. And nurses make up the largest part of this enormous organisation.

8

How to Influence Policy: Interviews with People Who Have

This final chapter presents an account of the work of three key UK nurses who have influenced the profession and policy for nursing in significant ways. My aim is to present positive role models although the chapter does not draw back from discussing the difficulty of their work and some of the trade-offs that they are forced to make in order to win certain policy battles – as that is obviously part of being an effective leader. I have interviewed Dr Peter Carter, the present General Secretary of the Royal College of Nursing, Dame Christine Beasley, recently retired Chief Nurse for England and Jane Salvage, prominent nurse intellectual and former head of nursing in Europe for the World Health Organization. In the interviews we focussed on the particular influence they have had and discussed key features of successful influencing. I finish the chapter with an up-beat summary of nursing's contribution to contemporary health care and speculation, from these three leaders, about its future. I finish the book with an ode to criticality – musical score to be supplied at a later date.

In the previous chapter we thought about health policy and discovered its complexity, its blend of ideology and science, the powerful interest groups involved and the high public visibility of health care in the United Kingdom. In this chapter I start not with structures but with individuals. I want to explore three things: the career trajectory and decisions of prominent nurse leaders, how they have set about trying to influence policy themselves and how they see a positive future for UK nursing.

Christine Beasley was England's Chief Nurse in the English Department of Health[1] from 2004 and retired in 2012, having delayed this at least once at the request of the Department. I interviewed her in her office in Richmond House in early 2012 and the recording is punctuated by the chimes of Big Ben. She started nursing in 1962 at the London Hospital and after qualifying moved in to community nursing jobs. She cut her teeth managing NHS organisations in both the community and acute sectors where changes, restructures and financial stringencies were ongoing. In the 1980s and early 1990s she took on senior roles at Ealing Health Authority and Riverside Health Authorities, both in west London, before moving into regional nurse director posts at North Thames Regional Health Authority (which no longer exists). She said that her NHS management posts taught her, among other things, how to work with trade unions during times of strife by establishing common ground.

She was awarded an Honorary Doctorate in nursing from Thames Valley University in 1997 and made a DBE (Dame Commander of the Order of the British Empire) in the queen's birthday honours in 2008. She has been one of the award presenters at Nursing Standard's Nurse of the Year ceremonies for at least the last 2 years, and on the most recent occasion (2012) she asked, with a grin, to be invited back in 2013, after her retirement, so that she could speak freely about her views on nursing and its place in government health policy. She has been Chief Nurse in England during some of the most testing times for the profession in terms of its public reputation.

Jane Salvage describes herself as a policy activist and compared to the other key influencers interviewed, her career and her mode of influence are more varied.[2] She was an English literature graduate

---

[1] The other countries of the United Kingdom have their own government chief nurses. Since Christine's retirement, the nursing voices at the Department of Health and NHS are represented by Viv Bennett and Jane Cummings, respectively. Jane Cummings works on the NHS Commissioning Board.

[2] The summary of her career comes partly from Nursing Times.net Hall of Fame at http://www.nursingtimes.net/whats-new-in-nursing/hall-of-fame/jane-salvage-empowered-nurses-in-the-uk-and-internationally/5012109.article and partly from her interview.

who then chose to train as a nurse. While a student nurse she was offered a regular column in *Nursing Mirror* which she used to critically comment on what she experienced at work, to the annoyance of her employer. The director of education of her hospital school of nursing asked her at one point to submit any writing to her for prior approval (an early indication that nursing is not necessarily one big happy family, with some senior nurses having an ambivalent approach to the public discussion of problems). Jane refused. After a number of years working as a staff nurse, she was offered a full-time job as journalist with *Nursing Mirror*, with training thrown in.

Eventually she became editor-in-chief of *Nursing Times*, a post she held from 1996 to 2001. Jane also was regional adviser for nursing and midwifery at the Regional Office for Europe, World Health Organization, 1991–1995, and director of the Nursing Developments Programme, King's Fund, 1988–1991. These roles involved her in developing nursing policy and practice in the United Kingdom and overseas.

Among her many publications, Jane is best known for her first book, *The Politics of Nursing*, published in 1985 by Heinemann. The main intention of the book was to raise the political consciousness of practising nurses – the profession's tendency to silence and somnambulism, according to Jane, its worst aspects. Journalism is only one strand of Jane's work around nursing policy. She worked in the secretariats and drafted the reports of both the Prime Minister's Commission on the Future of Nursing and Midwifery in England (2010)[3] and the Willis Commission on Nursing Education (2012). At the time of writing, she is a visiting professor at the Florence Nightingale School of Nursing and Midwifery, King's College London, and works as an independent consultant.

Peter Carter became General Secretary and Chief Executive Office of the Royal College of Nursing in 2007. He followed the

---

[3] This was set up by then Prime Minister Gordon Brown in 2009 and reported shortly before the Labour government lost power. Its aims were to create a long-term vision for the future of nursing and recommend some ways forward. Perhaps largely because of the change of government, the Commission did not realise its potential in as far as shaping the terms of debate about nursing. This could also be seen as further evidence that nursing is not a policy priority for governments.

rather unpopular and sometimes controversial Beverley Malone who had been in post from 2001. Before joining one of the world's largest professional union of nurses,[4] like many of the RCN's previous leaders, Peter had a career in NHS management. His entry into nursing was as a mental health nurse, and later he worked in an adolescent unit in St. Albans, north of London. He says that dealing with disturbed adolescents was a good preparation for working with some politicians and other challenging figures in his career. He has an MBA from the University of Birmingham and is a graduate and member of the Chartered Institute of Personnel and Development.

Preamble: Leadership and communication

If leadership is largely about influencing, then communication is a significant aspect of leadership. Added to this, today's political figures, people in public office, are under intense scrutiny from those in whose interests it could be to present them badly either because they are political opponents or because it could make a good story. Problems, conflict, scandal, inconsistency of message, apparent weakness are all emphasised or conjured up by the media, to such an extent that political discourse in many countries appears to be largely an exercise in avoiding embarrassments rather than setting out strategy. The leader of the United Kingdom's largest nursing trade union and the Chief Nurse are likely to be only too aware of this.

How does the career of a leader start?

Just like the rest of us, these leaders seemed to have had no master plan for their careers, and sometimes were unable to give detailed reasons for their career choices and trajectories. Peter Carter and Chris Beasley took up nursing in their teens.

---

[4] The RCN was first expanded to include certain categories of healthcare support workers in 2001. Nearly all HCSWs were able to join from 2005, and from 2011 they were permitted to become full members.

I didn't have this vision that I wanted to be a psychiatric nurse; I, at 18, didn't have a clue what I wanted to do and I bumped into an old school friend and he said he was training to be a psychiatric nurse and I said, what's that and he told me about it and . . . I absolutely loved it, I absolutely loved it. None of my family had ever been nurses or doctors or physios and I didn't even know what a psychiatric hospital was, fell into it and absolutely embraced it.

(Peter)

I trained at the London, now the Royal London Hospital, Whitechapel, so that's where I started my nursing career and I guess I was one of those little girls who always wanted to be a nurse although there was no medical history in the family and, in a way, what I thought I wanted to do when I was younger stayed with me although I looked up other careers and I suppose the reason why I wanted to nurse in those days was, I was very attracted to doing something working with people – I think that's what attracted me and when I was young careers were slightly more limited in the numbers of choices that you had. I came back into nursing [after bringing up my children] almost by accident – and anyway . . . I fell into district nursing almost by chance.

(Christine)

Jane Salvage had other life experiences before turning to nursing and had also experienced the death of her younger brother Guy. Her account of her motives for entering nursing is complex:

My path into nursing was unusual. I did an English Literature degree at Cambridge so going into nursing was not something that most people from there did and was seen by some people as a waste of a good education. But for me at the time, it was a mixture of reasons and many of them weren't accessible at the time and it's only later that I've come to understand . . . and I think there was a conscious sense I had that firstly, being involved in this was a very authentic and worthwhile thing to do; secondly, a lot of the things I experienced and my family experienced during my brother's death in hospital were very poorly handled I think, so I had a desire to put that right.

(Jane)

While Peter Carter and Christine Beasley speak of loving 'every minute of it' and 'absolutely loving it', Jane Salvage spoke of coming to nursing and immediately finding herself in an uncomfortable situation:

It felt right away that where I was and who I was, I was just like a cuckoo in the nest of nursing; I just felt very out of place. I was out of place anyway because I was in the graduate set, so I was with 11 others who were doing the shortened 2-year, 3-month course for registration so it meant we were separate, we were resented because we were doing a shorter course and there were lots of assumptions about being clever–clever and all sorts of fantasies about what having a degree meant. We all at one time or another wanted to leave. We all had a very similar critique of it being that we were infantilised, that it was like being back at school and the kind of approach that we'd experienced at university just was still not happening in the School of Nursing.

(Jane)

All three moved on from their entry to nursing, Christine Beasley and Peter Carter to management posts, though taking different routes, while Jane Salvage moved on from being a practitioner to other roles. Christine's story of her move into increasingly high profile management posts relied, in her account, repeatedly on two factors: being urged by more senior figures to apply and her decision to 'move out of my comfort zone'.

So somebody who'd been a divisional nurse had said to me . . . you should be thinking about doing something different, you shouldn't be staying in [this organisation] and I was comfortable in Ealing [in west London], I knew everybody and I liked my job and those things, but I did then begin to think well, do I really want to be doing this in the next 10 years? . . . So again, I guess, it was a good lesson around people who urge you on to do other things. Certainly, I've tried to do that as I've had people working for me to learn those lessons.

(Christine)

Peter Carter's account features more self-direction and the gathering of formal qualifications:

[In] my late 20s, I realised that I didn't want to do it [ward nursing] for the rest of my life. Even though I loved it and embraced it, and then I just went off and did other things and then eventually –

M: For instance?
P: Oh, I went off into managerial roles, I also I went to night school and I put myself into night school and did the Chartered Institute of Personnel and Development and I loved finding out about organisational behaviour and I did a lot of statistics and it got me into a world that I'd previously not been in at all. And then I embarked onto a management career, and then went to university – I did an MBA and I did my PhD and I ended up being a Chief Executive of a large NHS Trust here in London, which I did for 12 years and really enjoyed it. (Peter)

After qualifying, Jane Salvage was given opportunities that, in her words, were too good to turn down. Much of her subsequent career involved acting on nursing, sometimes with a formal position inside its professional structures, and sometimes outside these.

I started writing about what I was experiencing so I sent in an article about the [hospital] cuts in East London to a nursing magazine and, to my amazement, they published [it] . . . They then invited me to do a regular column – it was Nursing Mirror – so I had a student nurse soapbox column . . . I got through the training and then worked as a staff nurse for a while . . . but then I was thinking maybe I wanted to leave the hospital and do some heath visiting or something that would be more community based and just at that point where I wasn't sure what I wanted to do, I was offered a full time job by Nursing Mirror which meant going there and having a training in journalism as I was doing the job and it was too good to turn down and, in fact, that meant that I never returned to full time clinical nursing from then.

(Jane)

Influencing

I was interested in how these three leaders approached influencing the profession. All were differently placed and might be expected to influence in different ways. As people who might be considered to have the leading positions in nursing in England and the United Kingdom, Christine Beasley and Peter Carter might be expected to exercise a great deal of personal power; however, ironically, influencing for them involved a great deal of pragmatism and working within constraints. Christine's modus operandi recalled Strong and Robinson's picture of nursing as low down on the policy agenda (Strong and Robinson 1990):

I think from a nursing perspective, for good or ill, it's very hard to get nursing right up in the front as the driving force, it's hard – it's only right up in the front when they're all moaning about it and it's all bad. So what I learnt about it was that you saw what the strategic direction [of policy] was going to be ... and then think right, how do I hook the nursing agenda – I don't mean how do you bend the nursing agenda but how do I ride and not be too proud about that because ... you just have to say, hey, that's the way life is ... So I learned how to do that; I learned how to spot policies, I learned how to make alliances, I learned how to make partnerships with other folk – sometimes clinical, sometimes general managers and also learn how to say, actually, you know, nurses are such a big workforce – if we somehow don't impact on them, you're never going to get this [policy] to work.

One opportunity that presented itself was the previous New Labour administration's interest in nursing, under Secretary of State Alan

Milburn. Partly, Christine said, the reasons were a simple need to respond to the European working hours directive that reduced the hours worked by junior doctors. But partly, as I've discussed in previous chapters, Milburn wanted, like many predecessors in the Department of Health, to curtail the power of medicine. Nursing could be drawn into this strategy with ease by offering the professional attractions of policy attention around new roles and, in particular, the abilities to prescribe medicines:

> [the government realised that] nurses had a significant contribution to make ... and of course, they'd started to take on wider roles as well because of all the junior doctors [hours reduction] ... And then I think the thing that was less edifying is that they were keen to break the cartel of the doctors and this was a way of doing it. When I first got into this post, we were in the tail end of trying to push through nurse prescribing ... and the reason the BMA [British Medical Association] and others opposed it so vociferously was because it was the last hurdle that separated doctors from everybody. It opened up work.

Christine pointed out that a change of government, or even change of minister, can result in abruptly changed agendas, with work on particular initiatives coming to a complete stop. She also spoke, perhaps optimistically, of the importance of respecting the democratic mandate that governments possessed to make the changes they wished. The role of civil servants is to facilitate the work of ministers, and the work of ministers is legitimate because their parties are voted into office.

> It is also about being a civil servant, so you do get into the bit about you are here to serve, to serve intelligently, not just passively, the democratically elected government of the day and that is the job. They do have a mandate. People may not like the mandate. People may think they didn't vote for them, but our system is that it is legitimate for them to say here we are, we were voted in. So I think you have to keep that in your mind and if you can't live with that, you can't be a civil servant. That doesn't mean it's

unthinking because I've never worked with a minister that doesn't expect civil servants to challenge as well as to agree.

Christine pointed to two possible sources of frustration for the prospective strategic planner. The first concerned how politicians determined policy priorities. The particular skill of politicians, in Christine's view, was their ability to find the issues that their constituents felt were priorities and to use this intelligence to drive policy formation. This had the potential effect of skewing priorities away from those which an informed insider might consider important. The second, and linked, factor concerned the issues that the media emphasised at any particular point in time. According to Christine, there was often a 5-year time lag in this coverage, giving the impression that an issue, such as hospital acquired infection, was still a key threat when, in fact, it had been already largely dealt with.

Returning to the matter of pragmatism and influence, Christine felt strongly that the would-be influencer who held an official position needed a particular kind of approach, or personality:

> So it's a slightly pragmatic approach to it really and I suppose that's why I'm here; I mean, I'm not a revolutionary because you'd need a different tactic and I often say to people … if you want to be a revolutionary, being in here isn't the place for you to be because it will kill you … If you want to be a revolutionary, you need to be somewhere else … I think it's good to have revolutionaries and to have people challenging the system but they've got to be outside the system pushing it because you often have to do very uncomfortable things that are not always easy. So that doesn't mean to say you don't have any principles and you can't do anything within the system. I suppose the really effective thing is to be able to link some of that and what people can do and then you can really make some change.

Peter Carter also foregrounded the constraints that he was under as the leader of an organisation that needed to show accountability

to its members. On the one hand it was possible to exercise so
leadership:

> You have to come to terms with the fact that, at any given time,
> there will be people that fundamentally disagree with you. Ok,
> there's that. The other thing which you have to work out is that
> with a membership of 420,000 people, it is virtually impossible to
> be connecting with everybody's agenda but every day, the postbag
> is huge . . . we make sure that we answer every query, often giving
> people the answer to things that they don't want to hear. But it's
> important to be very straight with the membership.

It was also possible to take a stand that he knew would be unpopular
among members. Peter gave the example of not opposing the public sector pay freeze announced by the coalition government soon
after it came to power. But like Christine Beasley, his reasons were
pragmatic:

> So I made that decision and I got some stick for it, people wrote,
> 'you're gutless', you're this, that and the other, but equally, when
> I was going out – I'd go all over the country -- when I do meetings
> like this, most people were saying they thought that was right;
> they thought that was the politically astute, pragmatic thing to
> do – it was a fight we couldn't win.

On the other hand he spoke of failing to receive a mandate from
RCN members for action against changes to the nurses' pension
scheme to be imposed by the government. The RCN balloted its
members:

> only 16% [voted]. And remember, of the people that voted, it was
> 60% basically voted to reject the deal but nearly 40% voted to
> accept it. So then . . . what do we do with this? We have a tiny
> percentage of the membership voting and, of that tiny percent-
> age, 40% are actually saying they want to accept the deal. So our
> view is that the game's up; we're going to have to accept these

proposals. So, if people say to me, well, you're giving up the fight, I say, no, I'm not giving up the fight – you didn't give us the ammunition that we needed to go back to the government.

Jane Salvage's career has involved a great deal of policy work. Here she talks about the way she has used journalism to influence:

> I wrote about things that I thought needed to be changed, so it seemed to me that it was a fantastic platform for encouraging change, encouraging debate; the sort of debate that just didn't seem to be going on, apart from small radical pockets... For me part of it's about never forgetting what people are actually doing, having an understanding of what it feels like to be the health visitor in Newham or a staff nurse. Throughout my career, I've tried always to look at things from that standpoint. Nursing Times is a mass circulation magazine for an incredibly diverse group of people but you've always got to remember who they are and it's no good writing high-falutin' articles that are going to pass everybody by; they're busy people, they don't have a lot of time for reading.

Her motivation has not always been primarily to further a specific agenda but to have an effect on the consciousness of nurses and the consciousness of others such as the public and politicians about nursing issues as, in her own words, a policy activist:

> I always felt that nurses did not see themselves as having any influence over policy apart from a very small number in the top, so called, jobs like the CNO [Chief Nursing Officer] or head of the RCN, so I suppose part of my mission has been to encourage nurses to think that they can and should have a voice in decisions that are made about what their future might hold and how they do their work... whether it's ward policy, hospital policy, government policy... I think a lot of it's about encouraging people to find their voices, rather than me saying I've got the solution.

Jane described a situation without the constraint that formal office might have brought:

The first time I ever did a speech about nursing, I was inv...
to make a speech at the RCN students' association conferenc...
I'd never done anything quite like that before but it was on th...
back of my columns, so they wanted a controversial speaker. I just
stood up there and said what I thought, with some trepidation,
and what I've always found is when I've spoken from my truth, it
speaks to other people – not everyone of course – but I always get
people coming up and saying I'm so glad you said that because it's
what I'm thinking but I haven't been able, willing or courageous
enough to say.

Nursing's number one issue

When I asked what my interviewees thought was the most important
current issue for nursing, there was consensus that the profession
was at a crossroads of reputation and self-direction:

> The over-arching [topic] right now is the issue of, the perception
> of nursing having falling from a pedestal, that nurses give poor
> care and the apparent loss of public trust in nursing, to the extent
> that Private Eye even has a cartoon called 'Fallen Angels'.
>
> (Jane)

> For me, the biggest issue ... is the image of nursing. Over the last
> year or two, there has been a steady stream of very unfavourable
> reports on standards.
>
> (Peter)

Christine Beasley feared that nursing's current bad press, along with
continuing turbulence at the NMC (discussed in Chapter 3), might
open the way for politicians to aim the 'magic bullet' of a quick fix in
the profession's direction, and in the process rob it of autonomy and
undo some of its recent gains:

> There is no doubt about it, there are areas where we let down our
> public population – it isn't just the odd nurse in the odd ward.
> So some of it, we can't be getting right ... [but] what politicians

...ant is any sort of quick answer to the problem. What I find difficult and I still struggle with, is recognising that politically, they have to be seen to be doing something. These magic bullets [such as]: 'if only we didn't educate nurses, if only nurses were more stupid' – nursing is the only profession where being more intelligent is seen as some sort of hindrance. It goes from that to maybe 'if they wore uniforms'; if you did this, if you did that like a magic bullet that would make a difference . . . they're so driven by wanting it to be made right.

Peter Carter agreed that there were spurious explanations for this nursing 'failure' circulating in the media:

There's this myth around that the trouble is because [nurses are] all degree educated. Well, that's an absolute myth partly, because, statistically speaking, most nurses actually don't have a degree so if you attribute all the ills to the fact that they're all degree educated, that doesn't stand up to scrutiny. But I still don't under-stand where the mind-set comes in that – if you've got a degree, that you can't be caring. I mean, there is no logic to that all.

(Peter)

He believed that a more likely explanation lay in a health system that had failed to adapt to and invest for an ageing population:

There's a mind-set that when you're looking after older people, all you need is a bit of common sense and some tender loving care. Well you need those qualities but you need a heck of a lot more so when you get these accounts of relatives saying, 'well we came to visit mum and it was clear she hadn't had a drink or she'd been incontinent and they hadn't cleaned her up'. I don't believe that those staff are wilfully negligent; I believe it's because they're working in systems which are virtually impossible to.

Christine felt that claims of understaffing could not account for poor care alone. Rather it could be the relentlessness of work

in emotionally demanding environments, without the reward
patients regularly improving and going home, that could desensiti·
workers.

Jane identified part of the problem as an incompatibility between
modern healthcare systems and nursing ideology:

> [there is] this enormous pressure [of patient throughput] and at
> the same time the ideal that everybody should be cared for in
> a way that we've learned to describe nursing in the last 20–30
> years – the holistic way where you're providing the full spectrum
> of care ranging from – heaven help us – spiritual care, care around
> sexuality right through. So this amazingly – I almost want to say,
> over-weening – but an extraordinarily ambitious sense of what it is
> that we're doing when we're looking after somebody . . . Inevitably
> we always fall short and then we can beat ourselves up about it
> and be beaten up by everybody else for being failures as nurses.

My respondents were aware of the myth of a wonderful past for
nursing, and all felt that this was unhelpful and basically inaccu-
rate. Christine is talking about the misguided ambitions of some
politicians:

> If [politicians] could take nursing back to what they think was the
> golden age of nursing where nurses were in hospitals in a nursing
> school, you know, that on the whole were nice women being kind,
> they would do it, but they can't.

Jane elaborated on why she believed there was no 'golden age'. For
her the impression of a current crisis in nursing is being fuelled
partly by a more active, investigative media and partly by the rise
in regulatory bodies, as discussed in Chapter 7, rising throughput
and spiralling demand for ever more complex care:

> I think it's a very interesting question whether it actually is any
> worse than it was before and there's no way of knowing but
> certainly fantasies of the golden age where everything was just

wonderful are just that and my memories of clinical nursing are that terrible things happened but they were covered up or you didn't even realise they were terrible...there wasn't the focus on measurement of quality – a different kind of focus on quality perhaps – but lots of abuse, active abuse or neglect – we can all remember lots of examples.

(Jane Salvage)

A positive future for nursing

Finally I wanted to know how these three leading figures saw nursing in an ideal future. I had the impression that, given their heavy day-to-day involvement in grappling with the reality of situations rather than discussing ideal states, they would have benefitted from more time to refocus and consider their answers. Nevertheless their responses reflected the positions that each spoke from. All of their answers had today's reality woven into their vision. Christine talked first about the route that the profession would need to take to get to a better future:

> There are some big issues about nursing owning itself and taking responsibility...not either being passive, which is very easy for nurses to be, or slightly denying [the recent problems] or saying it's only because we haven't got enough nurses. That may be some of the case, but actually, all poor care doesn't happen in places where there aren't enough staff, if only that was just the issue...

She went on to describe a possible future for nursing:

> I think it would be building on all the good things we've got to build on so that individual nurses are having very satisfying careers. There's a good platform for that in terms of what I think, education [can offer], things that you can do, whether it's technical things like prescribing, all those sorts of things to enhance your skills or if you're a mental health nurse, it's the recovery approach. There's some real opportunities to make fantastic interventions on that level...and I think a greater recognition about

what nursing can contribute...There are lots of very positive things I think about nursing and I think it is still a fantastic career to be involved in. Some of the challenges [are] that we as nurses have got to start talking up the profession – I don't mean in an unrealistic, 'it's marvellous', sort of way.

For Christine innovative and intelligent service development was at the heart of the potential she saw in nursing. She gave examples of individual services around England that she had visited where nurses had developed ways of working that seemed to improve patient experience, outcomes and make nursing work more interesting and rewarding.

Jane's approach started from the perspective of the individual nurse and then moved on to acknowledge the kind of system change required to make this fantasy possible.

My fantasy has always been what I wanted for myself when I was nursing which was to be able to be that holistic practitioner; to be able to care wonderfully for someone who's going to love me because I care wonderfully for them, then I go home with this wonderful sense of satisfaction that I've really made a difference, a positive difference, to someone, which you do feel in nursing sometimes. I've always wanted to be able to create the conditions for myself and others to be able to give that kind of care, to have that kind of satisfaction, not to be exhausted all the time, not to be chastised all the time, obviously to be able to learn and do things better and to learn from mistakes, but actually, just to do this brilliant job.

However, drawing on her own experience of nursing her mother, her vision extended to more structural change:

I still believe in all the things we've talked about so much over the years about trying to shift the whole emphasis of the [health] system towards prevention, public health. Nurses' involvement in public health and community care to be much greater, where much more care is given at home, where people with long term conditions will be able to stay at home and get the support that they need.

Pay and conditions are the core business of a trade union, and Peter Carter's opening comments reflect this. In a sense he would be failing in his role if he were to ignore this in a consideration of an ideal future for nursing. However he quickly moved on to a defence of degree-level qualification for nurses (a recurrent theme in this book). In one sense this is a less predictable response for someone speaking from Peter's position. Of course the status and rewards given to nurses are, at least in part, dependent on their level of preparation, and advances in education are a core part of any professionalising project. However, the profession has been chronically divided on this issue, and if the whole membership of the RCN did turn out to vote on what they thought about this topic, the result may not be as progressive as Peter's commitment.

I know some people are going to say, it's not about money and I know it's not about money but realistically, people are doing very difficult jobs and I actually do think pay is very important. I think that people are worth more: ward sisters, 36 grand – it's absurd. I know I started with pay but I just wanted to get that out of the way. But what I would hope would have settled down is this mythology that they're too well educated, too posh to wash, too clever to care; all these headlines that you see that we'll have worked through that, and people will have understood that the evolving nature of nursing is such that you need well educated people, that a degree is something you should be proud about.

Peter, like others in his post before him, and echoing Jane Salvage, wished for a nursing workforce that was far more politically engaged. Again, like many other activists in nursing, he was pained by the contradiction between the size of the workforce and the low confidence and little influence that the profession wielded:

What my dream is, is that nurses find more time to get politically engaged with both a capital and a small p. ... I'd like to think that nurses would begin to realise that you're a huge discipline, you've got a huge amount of muscle power, political power, but there's something in the DNA of nurses that we don't kind of realise it in the way that so many other disciplines do.

Some final thought experiments

Do you agree with these three leaders about the causes of nurses giving poor care i.e. a mixture of inadequate resources and unrealistic expectations about what a nurse can do? From your own experience, would you add other factors?

They wished for a future where nurses had higher satisfaction, more pay, were creating innovative services and were more involved in policy decisions. As someone with a future in nursing ahead of you, what else would you add to this vision?

Christine and Peter were adamant that moving to degree-level entry to nursing was a positive move and disagreed with those who claimed that this has led to a workforce who are less inclined to care. What is your view about this? If you have had contact with colleagues with and without degree-level qualification, would you say there are systematic differences between them?

If you were appointed Chief Nurse, what would be the first two initiatives you would set in motion?

Finale: Context is everything – nothing is innocent

If you have read this book from the beginning, congratulations on reaching the end of this final chapter. The main intention of the book has been to discuss issues that nurses have to deal with on a daily basis in a realistic way, free from the confusion between idealised versions of how things should be and how they actually are.

This book is an attempt to provide concepts, theories and a language that you can use to disassemble the forces and arguments acting upon nursing in health care and society at large. Each chapter has focussed on one part of an interrelated matrix of policy, political and professional issues: nursing's history and its present identity, education for practice, professional regulation and its ambiguities, nursing's place in the healthcare division of labour, the evidence-based movement and the authority of research, nursing in health policy and approaches to influencing it, and the complex spectacle of failures of care. A sustained examination, which I hope this book has provided, reveals that there is more to these, and other issues, than meets the eye. Many assumptions upon which action has been based, regarding so-called poor performance to take just one example, do not stand up to scrutiny, yet actors put a great deal of effort into maintaining various collective fantasies in order to maintain sufficient stability to achieve a number of deeply unexamined goals.

A great many speeches, pamphlets, websites and books exhort nurses to do more: to put research into practice, to exercise leadership, to get involved in policy, to care, to innovate, to reflect on practice, to keep to the code, to blow the whistle, to not blow the whistle. These exhortations all seem to emerge from groups already committed to particular positions and projects wanting to further these with your support, energy and by you generally taking them seriously. Critical questioning about the overall goal or the underlying values or assumptions of these projects or practices is sometimes not welcomed by their proponents, not necessarily because there is some conspiracy but more often because people are under pressure, as this book has shown, and want things to go smoothly.

But the decision that basic nurse training take the form of a university degree represents an opportunity to raise the level of sophistication and criticality of our thought and action. Although some health service managers and senior nurses (and even educators) would perhaps secretly wish for a nursing workforce that is hard working and compliant rather than enquiring and questioning, the nurse education genie is out of the bottle now and with any luck it will not be returning.

The sophisticated and critical individual who can draw on a theoretical framework or on analytical habits of thought to understand their experiences in nursing, or in any other field, has a huge advantage over others. What started out feeling like a personal failure, the inability to provide a high standard of patient care for example, can turn out, with some analysis, to be the almost unavoidable, built-in result of a series of structural forces and prior decisions. So the advantage for the person who has developed criticality is increased confidence and a therapeutic benefit, both of which are immensely valuable in tough times. It may also equip that person to resist, challenge or push for change.

It is my hope that studying for a degree will enable nursing students to develop that criticality and that this book, by examining crucial issues for nurses, will in some way help towards that.

References

Abel-Smith, B. (1960). *A History of the Nursing Profession*. London, Heinemann Educational.

Allen, D. (1997). 'Studied Recommendations.' *Nursing Standard* **11**(45): 11.

Allen, D. (2001). *The Changing Shape of Nursing Practice: The Role of Nurses in the Hospital Division of Labour*. London, Routledge.

Allsop, J. and M. Saks, Eds. (2002). *Regulating the Health Professions*. London, Sage.

Atkinson, P., M. Reid, et al. (1977). 'Medical Mystique.' *Sociology of Work and Occupations* **4**(3): 243–280.

Baars, S. and ISC (University of Manchester) (2010). Social class, aspirations and cultural capital: a case study of working class children's plans for the future and their parents' involvement in life beyond the school gates. *ISC Working Paper 2010–05*. Manchester, Institute for Social Change, University of Manchester.

Barker, P. (2000). 'Commentaries and Reflections on Mental Health Nursing in the UK at the Dawn of a New Millennium: Commentary' *Journal of Mental Health* **9**: 617–619.

BBC News (2010). Majority of Young Women in University. Retrieved 10 December 2011, from http://news.bbc.co.uk/1/hi/education/8596504.stm.

BBC News (8 November 2010). 'Timeline: Stafford Hospital in Crisis 2007–2010.' Retrieved 4 February 2011, from http://news.bbc.co.uk/local/stoke/hi/people_and_places/newsid_8493000/8493964.stm.

BBC News Channel (2004). 'Women Docs "weakening" Medicine.' Retrieved 17 September 2011 from http://news.bbc.co.uk/1/hi/health/3527184.stm.

BBC Panorama (2009). 'Who'd Be a NHS Whistleblower?' Retrieved October 31 2011, from http://news.bbc.co.uk/panorama/hi/front_page/newsid_8014000/8014206.stm.

BBC Panorama (2011). 'Undercover Care: The Abuse Exposed.' Retrieved 9 June 2011, from http://www.bbc.co.uk/programmes/b011pwt6.

Becher, T. and M. Kogan (1992). *Process and Structure in Higher Education*. London, Routledge.

Beck, U. (1992). *Risk Society: Towards a New Modernity*. London, Sage.

Bellefontaine, N. (2009). 'Exploring Whether Student Nurses Report Poor Practice They Have Witnessed on Placements.' *Nursing Times* **105**(35): 28–31.

Bixler, G. K. and R. W. Bixler (1945). 'The Professional Status of Nursing.' *The American Journal of Nursing* **45**(9): 730–735.

Blumer, H. G. (1969). Collective Behavior. *Principles of Sociology*. A. McClung Lee (Ed.). New York, Barnes and Noble Books, 65–121.

BMJ (2005). 'UK Doctors Protest at Extension to Nurses' Prescribing Powers.' *BMJ* **331**(1159.1).

Bradley, E. and P. Nolan (2008). *Non-Medical Prescribing: Multi-Disciplinary Perspectives*. Cambridge, Cambridge University Press.

Bradshaw, A. (2009). 'Measuring Nursing Care and Compassion: The McDonaldised Nurse?' *Journal of Medical Ethics* **35**: 465–468.

Brown, C. (1997). 'Fees May be Waived for Medical Students.' *The Independent* 6th August: 6.

Carmel, S. (2003). High Technology Medicine in Practice: The Organisation of Work in Intensive Care. *Faculty of Medicine*. London, University of London (London School of Hygiene & Tropical Medicine), PhD.

Carvel, J. (2004). NHS Trust Reinstates Crouton Surgeon. *The Guardian*, London.

Carvel, J. and R. Allison (2001). Watchdog Says Hospital Waiting Lists Were Fiddled: Audit Office Says Patients Were Betrayed by Massaging of Figures. *The Guardian*, London.

CHRE (2011). *NMC Progress Review: A Review of the NMC's Fitness to Practise Directorate's Progress Since 2008*. London, Council For Healthcare Regulatory Excellence.

Committee on Nursing (1972). *Report of the Committee on Nursing (Chairman: Asa Briggs)*. Cmnd. 5115. London, HMSO.

Cooke, H. (2006). 'Examining the Disciplinary Process in Nursing: A Case Study Approach.' *Work Employment and Society* **20**(4): 687–707.

Cooke, H. (2012). Changing Discourses of Blame in Nursing and Healthcare. *(Re)Thinking Violence in Health Care Settings: A Critical Approach*. D. Holmes, T. Rudge and A. Perron (Eds). Farnham, Surrey, Ashgate, 47–66.

Care Quality Commission. (9 June 2011). 'Dignity and Nutrition Reports.' Retrieved 9 June 2011, from http://www.cqc.org.uk/newsandevents/newsstories.cfm?FaArea1=customwidgets.content_view_1&cit_id=37390.

Crisp, N. (2005). Commissioning a Patient-Led NHS, 28 July 2005 Gateway reference number: 5312. Department of Health, 10.

Cullum, N. (1997). 'Identification and Analysis of Randomised Controlled Trials in Nursing: A Preliminary Study.' *Quality in Health Care* **6**(1): 2–6.

Cullum, N., D. Ciliska, et al., Eds. (2008). *Evidence-Based Nursing. An Introduction*. Oxford, Blackwell and BMJ and RCN Publishing.

Currie, L. and Y. Richens (2009). 'Exploring the Perceptions of Midwifery Staff About Safety Culture.' *British Journal of Midwifery* **17**(12): 783–790.

Curtis, L. (2010). *Unit Costs of Health and Social Care 2010*. Canterbury, Personal Social Services Research Unit.

Davies, C. (1995). *Gender and the Professional Predicament in Nursing*. Buckingham, Open University Press.

Davies, C. (2002). What About the Girl Next Door? Gender and the Politics of Professional Self-Regulation. *Gender, Health and Healing: The Public/Private Divide*. G. Bendelow, M. Carpenter, C. Vautier and S. Williams (Eds). London, Routledge.

Davies, C. and A. Beach (2000). *Interpreting Professional Self-Regulation; A History of the United Kingdom Central Council for Nursing, Midwifery and Health Visiting.* London, Routledge.

Department for Education and Skills (2005). Has the social class gap narrowed in primary schools? Background note accompanying the talk by Rt Hon Ruth Kelly MP, Secretary of State for Education and Skills: "Education and Social Progress", 26 July 2005.

Department of Health (1989). *Working for Patients.* London, HMSO Cmd. 555.

Department of Health (1991). *Research for Health; A Research and Development Strategy for the NHS.* London, HMSO.

Department of Health (1997). *The New NHS; Modern Dependable.* London, Department of Health Cm 3807.

Department of Health (1999). *Making a Difference, Strengthening the Nursing, Midwifery and Health Visiting Contribution to Health and Healthcare.* London, Department of Health.

Department of Health (2000). *The NHS Plan: A Plan for Investment, a Plan for Reform.* London, Department of Health.

Department of Health. (14 November 2003). 'Nurses need to be all that they can be' – Reid.' Retrieved 1 November 2004, from http://www.dh.gov.uk/PublicationsAndStatistics/PressReleases/PressReleasesNotices/fs/en?CONTENT_ID=4062706&chk=7Y1%2Bpq.

Department of Health and CNO's Office (2006). *Modernising Nursing Careers – Setting the Direction.* London, Department of Health.

Department of Health and National Patient Safety Agency (2006). *Handling Concerns About the Performance of Healthcare Professionals: Principles of Good Practice.* London, NCAS.

Dingwall, R., A. M. Rafferty, et al. (1988). *An Introduction to the Social History of Nursing.* London, Routledge.

Draper, P. (1995). 'The Merger of United Kingdom Colleges of Nursing with Univeristy Departments of Nursing: Prospects, Problems and Promises.' *Journal of Advanced Nursing* **23**(3): 215–216.

Eagleton, T. (1983). *Literary Theory: An Introduction.* Oxford, Blackwell.

Elias, P. and K. Purcell (2004). Researching Graduate Careers Seven Years On: A Research Project Jointly Funded by the Economic and Social Research Council and the Higher Education Careers Services Unit. SOC (HE): A Classification of Occupations for Studying the Graduate Labour Market. Warwick, Employment Studies Research Unit, University of the West of England and Warwick Institute for Employment Research.

Etzioni, A., Ed. (1969). *The Semi-Professions and Their Organization.* New York, The Free Press.

Finn, R., M. Learmonth, et al. (2010). 'Some Unintended Effects of Teamwork in Healthcare.' *Social Science & Medicine* **70**(8): 1148–1154.

Firth-Cozens, J., R. Firth, et al. (2003). 'Attitudes to and Experiences of Reporting Poor Care.' *Clinical Governance: An International Journal* **8**(4): 331–336.

Fletcher, J. (1995). 'Snakes and Ladders: The Future of Nurse Education?' *Jour* *Nursing Management* **3**(1): 35–41.

Ford, S. (2012). 'Review Concludes NMC is Failing "at Every Level".' Retrieve 16 August 2012, from http://www.nursingtimes.net/nursing-practice/clinical-specialisms/management/review-concludes-nmc-is-failing-at-every-level/5046648. article.

Foucault, M. (1991). 'Governmentality,' trans. Rosi Braidotti and revised by Colin Gordon. *The Foucault Effect: Studies in Governmentality*. G. Burchell, C. Gordon and P. Miller (Eds). Chicago, IL, University of Chicago Press, 87–104.

Francis, R. (2010). *Final Report of the Independent Inquiry into Care Provided by Mid Staffordshire NHS Foundation Trust Published: Volume 1*. London, Stationery Office.

Freidson, E. (1970). *The Profession of Medicine: A Study of the Sociology of Applied knowledge*. Chicago Il., University of Chicago Press.

Freidson, E. (1994). *Professionalism Reborn*. Cambridge, Polity.

Furlong, A. (1993). *Schooling for Jobs: Changes in the Career Preparation of British Secondary School Children*. Aldershot, Ashgate Publishing.

Gabbay, J., A. Le May, et al. (2003). 'A Case Study of Knowledge Management in Multi-Agency Consumer-Informed 'Communities of Practice': Implications for Evidence-Based Policy Development in Health and Social Services.' *Health: An Interdisciplinary Journal for the Social Study of Health, Illness and Medicine* **7**(3): 283–310.

Giddens, A. (1990). *The Consequences of Modernity*. Cambridge, Polity Press.

Goldthorpe, J. H. (2003). 'The Myth of Education Based Meritocracy: Why the Theory isn't Working.' *New Economy* **10**(4): 234–239.

Gournay, K. (2000). 'Commentaries and Reflections on Mental Health Nursing in the UK at the Dawn of a New Millennium: Commentary 2.' *Journal of Mental Health* **9**: 621–623.

Green, H. and S. Parker (2006). *The Other Glass Ceiling: The Domestic Politics of Parenting*. London, DEMOS.

Griffiths, L. (1998). 'Humour as Resistance to Professional Dominance in Community Mental Health Teams.' *Sociology of Health & Illness* **20** (6): 874–895.

Harding Clark, M. (2006). The Lourdes Hospital Inquiry: An Inquiry into Peripartum Hysterectomy at Our Lady of Lourdes Hospital, Drogheda. Dublin.

Harrison, S. and W. Ahmad (2000). 'Medical Autonomy and the UK State 1975 to 2025.' *Sociology* **34**(1): 129–146.

Harrison, S. and C. Pollitt (1994). *Controlling Health Professionals; The Future of Work and Organisation in the NHS*. Buckingham, Open University Press.

Health Service Ombudsman. (2011). 'Report of the Health Service Ombudsman on ten Investigations into NHS Care of Older People.' Retrieved 9 June 2011, from http://www.ombudsman.org.uk/care-and-compassion.

Hek, G. and A. Shaw (2006). 'The Contribution of Research knowledge and Skills to Practice: An Exploration of the Views and Experiences of Newly Qualified Nurses.' *Journal of Research in Nursing* **11**(6): 473–482.

..s, C., D. Hennessy, et al. (1996). 'Investigating Attitudes to Research in Primary Health Care Teams.' *Journal of Advanced Nursing* **24**: 1033–1041.

..orton, R. (1995). 'Evidence-based Medicine, in its Place.' *Lancet* **346**(8978): 785.

Horton, R. (2002). 'Nurse-prescribing in the UK: Right But also Wrong.' *Lancet* **359** (9321): 1875–1876.

House of Lords Select Committee on Science and Technology (1988). *Priorities in Medical Research. 1st Report*. London, HMSO.

Hudson, P. (2011). 'Women's Work.' Retrieved from 18 September 2011 http://www.bbc.co.uk/history/british/victorians/womens_work_01.shtml.

ICN (1996). Better Health Through Nursing Research, International Council of Nurses.

Jamous, H. and B. Peloille (1970). Professions or Self-Perpetuating System; Changes in the French University-Hospital System. *Professions and Professionalisation*. J. Jackson. Cambridge, Cambridge University Press, 109–152.

JM Consulting Ltd. (1998). *The Regulation of Nurses, Midwives and Health Visitors*; Report on a Review of the Nurses, Midwives & Health Visitors Act 1997. Bristol, JM Consulting.

Johnson, D. (1974). 'Development of Theory: A Requisite for Nursing as a Primary Health Profession.' *Nursing Research* **23**(5): 372–377.

Karasek, R., C. Brisson, et al. (1998). 'The Job Content Questionnaire (JCQ): An Instrument for Internationally Comparative Assessments of Psychosocial Job Characteristics.' *Journal of Occupational Health Psychology* **4**(4): 322–355.

Katz, F. (1969). Nurses. *The Semi-Professions and Their Organization*. A. Etzioni. New York, The Free Press, 54–81.

Kavanagh, D. (2006). Pressure Groups and Policy Networks. *British Politics*. D. Kavanagh, D. Richards, A. Geddes and M. Smith (Eds). Oxford, Oxford University Press, 417–440.

Kennedy, I. and Bristol Royal Infirmary (2000). *The Inquiry into the Management of Care of Children Receiving Complex Heart Surgery at the Bristol Royal Infirmary*. Bristol, Central Office of Information.

Kennedy, I., Bristol Royal Infirmary Inquiry, et al. (2001). *Learning from Bristol: The Report of the Public Inquiry into Children's Heart Surgery at the Bristol Royal Infirmary 1984–1995*. Norwich, Stationery Office.

Kilminster, S., J. Downes, et al. (2007). 'Women in Medicine – Is There a Problem? A Literature Review of the Changing Gender Composition, Structures and Occupational Cultures in Medicine.' *Medical Education* **41**: 39–49.

Kitson, A. (1997). 'Using Evidence to Demonstrate the Value of Nursing.' *Nursing Standard* **11**(28): 34–39.

Koteyko, N. and B. Nerlich (2008). 'Modern Matrons and Infection Control Practices: Aspirations and Realities.' *British Journal of Infection Control* **9**(2): 18–22.

Laurance, J. (2004). Health Check: 'The Feminisation of the Medical Profession is Gathering Pace.' *The Independent on Sunday*. London.

Levine, L. (1863). *International Commercial Law: Being the Principles of Law of the Following and Other Countries, viz.: England, Scotland, Irelanc India, British Colonies, Austria, Belgium, Brazil, Buenos Ayres, Denmark, ι Germany, Greece, Hans Towns, Italy, Netherlands, Norway, Portugal, Prussia, Rι Spain, Sweden, Switzerland, United States, Wurtemburg.* London, V. and R. Stever Sons, and Haynes.

Light, D. (1995). Countervailing Powers. A Framework for Professions in Transition. *Health Professions and the State in Europe.* T. Johnson, G. Larkin and M. Saks (Eds). London, Routledge, 25–41.

Lomas, J. (1993). *Teaching Old (and not so old) Docs New Tricks: Effective Ways to Implement Research Findings.* Ontario, McMaster University Centre for Health Econmics and Policy Analysis.

May, C., V. M. Montori, et al. (2009). 'We Need Minimally Disruptive Medicine.' *BMJ* **2012**(August): 339:b2803.

McClarey, M. and L. Duff (1997). 'Clinical Effectiveness and Evidence-Based Practice.' *Nursing Standard* **11**(52): 33–35.

McGann, S. (1992). *The Battle of the Nurses: A Study of Eight Women Who Influenced the Development of Professional Nursing 1880–1930.* London, Scutari Press.

McKenna, H., S. Ashton, et al. (2004). 'Barriers to Evidence-Based Practice in Primary Care.' *Journal of Advanced Nursing* **45**(2): 178–189.

Meleis, A. (1985). *Theoretical Nursing: Development and Progress.* Philadelphia, J B Lippincott and Co.

Menzies, I. E. P. (1960). 'A Case Study in the Functioning of Social Systems as a Defence Against Anxiety: A Report on a Study of the Nursing Service of a General Hospital.' *Human Relations* **13**: 95–121.

Mickan, S. and S. Rodger (2005). 'Effective Health Care Teams: A Model of Six Characteristics Developed from Shared Perceptions.' *Journal of Interprofessional Care* **19**(4): 358–370.

Miers, M. E., C. E. Rickaby, et al. (2007). 'Career Choices in Health Care: Is Nursing a Special Case? A Content Analysis of Survey Data.' *International Journal of Nursing Studies* **44**(7): 1196–1209.

National Audit Office (1992). *Nursing Education.* Implementation of Project 2000 in England, Report by the Comptroller and Auditor General, HMSO.

National Clinical Assessment Service (2010). *Handling Performance Concerns in Primary Care: An NCAS Guide to Good Practice.* London, National Patient Safety Agency.

National Committee of Inquiry into Higher Education (1997). *Higher Education in the Learning Society; the Dearing Report.* London, Department of Education and Employment.

Naylor, C. D. (1995). 'Grey Zones of Clinical Practice: Some Limits to Evidence-Based Medicine.' *Lancet* **346**: 840–842.

Neilson, G. (2008). School Leavers into Nursing: A Study of High Academic Achieving School Pupils in Scottish Schools. *Education,* Stirling. Doctorate of Education, 432.

ɔ. and W. Lauder (2008). 'What Do High Academic Achieving School
. Really Think About a Career in Nursing: Analysis of the Narrative From
.digmatic Case Interviews.' *Nurse Education Today* **28**: 680–690.

ɔon, S. (1995). 'Humanism in Nursing: The Emergence of the Light.' *Nursing Inquiry* **2**(1): 36–43.

NHS Education for Scotland (2010). *The Development of the Clinical Healthcare Support Worker Role: A Review of the Evidence*. Edinburgh, NES.

NHS Institute for Innovation and Improvement and Royal College of Nursing (2007). *Developing and Sustaining Effective Teams*. London, RCN.

NMC (2008). *The Code: Standards of Conduct, Performance and Ethics for Nurses and Midwives*. London, Nursing and Midwifery Council.

NMC. (31 May 2011). 'NMC Comment on Panorama's Undercover Care: The Abuse Exposed.' Retrieved 9 June 2011, from http://www.nmc-uk.org/Press-and-media/Latest-news/NMC-comment-on-Panoramas-Undercover-Care-The-Abuse-Exposed/.

NMC_Admin (12 October 2011). 'Healthcare Regulation Explained.' Retrieved 5 February 2012, from http://www.nmc-review.org/issues/issue-3-autumn-w/understanding-regulation/box-1-healthcare-regulation-explained/.

Nursing and Midwifery Council (2009). *Fitness to Practise Annual Report 1 April 2008 to 31 March 2009*. London, NMC.

Nursing and Midwifery Council (2010). *Standards for Pre-Registration Nursing Education*. London, NMC, 152.

Nursing and Midwifery Council (2011). *Fitness to Practise Annual Report 2010–2011*. London, NMC, 27.

Nursing Standard News (1997). 'Nursing Students to Get Tuition Fees Paid.' *Nursing Standard* **12**(2): 5.

O'Malley, P. (2009). *The Sage Dictionary of Policing*. A. Wakefield and J. Fleming (Eds). London, Sage, 276–277.

Paley, J. (2006). 'Evidence and Expertise.' *Nursing Inquiry* **13**(2): 82–93.

Paterson, J. and L. Zderard (1976). *Humanistic Nursing*. New York, John Wiley.

Peters, T. and R. Waterman (1982). *In Search of Excellence*. New York, Harper and Row.

Pinder, R., R. Petchey, et al. (2005). 'What's in a Care Pathway? Towards a Cultural Cartography of the New NHS.' *Sociology of Health & Illness* **27**(6): 759–779.

Prime Minister's Commission (2010). *Front Line Care: Report by the Prime Minister's Commission on the Future of Nursing and Midwifery in England*. London, Department of Health.

Rafferty, A. M. (1996). *The Politics of Nursing Knowledge*. London, Routledge.

RCN. (26 May 2011). 'RCN Response to CQC Report on Dignity and Nutrition for Older People.' Retrieved 9 June 2011, from http://www.rcn.org.uk/newsevents/press_releases/uk/rcn_response_to_cqc_report_on_dignity_and_nutrition_for_older_people2.

Redmayne, S. (1995). *Reshaping the NHS; Strategies, Priorities and Resource* cation. London, Centre for the Analysis of Social Policy, University of Bath and National Association of Health Authorities and Trusts.

Reverby, S. (1987). 'A Caring Dilemma: Womanhood and Nursing in Historical Perspective.' *Nursing Research* **36**(1): 5–11.

Rivett, G. (2011). 'National Health Service History: 1998–2007 Labour's Decade.' Retrieved 15 August 2012, from http://www.nhshistory.net/chapter_6.html – Nursing.

Robinson, J. (1997). Power, Politics and Policy Analysis in Nursing. *Nursing: A Knowledge Base for Practice*. A. Perry (Ed.). London, Arnold, 249–281.

Robinson, J. and R. Elkan (1992). *Policy Issues in Nursing*. Milton Keynes, Open University Press.

Robinson, S. and J. Bennett (2007). *Career Choices and Constraints: Influences on Direction and Retention in Nursing*. London, King's College London, Nursing Research Unit.

Rognstad, M. K. and O. Aasland (2007). 'Change in Career Aspirations and Job Values From Study Time to Working Life.' *Journal of Nursing Management* **15**(4): 424–432.

Ross, F. (2010). 'Poor Organisational Cultures Erode Compassionate Care.' Retrieved 3 December 2011, from http://www.nursingtimes.net/poor-organisational cultures-erode-compassionate-care/5018269.article.

Royal College of Nursing (1996). *A Principled Approach to Nurse Education. The Rationale. A Document for Discussion*. London, RCN.

Royal College of Nursing (2003). *Defining Nursing*. London, RCN.

Sackett, D., W. Rosenberg, et al. (1996). 'Evidence-Based Medicine: What it is and What it isn't.' *British Medical Journal* **312**: 71–72.

Sackett, D. L. (1997). *Evidence-Based Medicine. How to Practice and Teach EBM*. New York, Churchill Livingstone.

Sackett, D. L. (2000). *Evidence-based Medicine: How to Practice and Teach EBM*. Edinburgh; New York, Churchill Livingstone.

Salhani, D. and I. Coulter (2009). 'The Politics of Interprofessional Working and the Struggle for Professional Autonomy in Nursing.' *Social Science & Medicine* **68**: 1221–1228.

Sartre, J.-P. (1957). Existentialism is a Humanism Written: Lecture Given in 1946. *Existentialism from Dostoyevsky to Sartre*. W. Kaufman (Ed.). London, Meridian Books, Thames and Hudson.

Savage, J. and C. Scott (2004). 'The Modern Matron: A Hybrid Management Role with Implications for Continuous Quality Improvement.' *Journal of Nursing Management* **12**(6): 419–426.

Seers, K. (1997). 'Editorial: Randomised Controlled Trials in Nursing.' *Quality in Health Care* **6**(1): 1.

Simpson, A. (2007). 'The Impact of Team Processes on Psychiatric Case Management.' *Journal of Advanced Nursing* **60**(4): 409–418.

...s for Health (2010). *The Role of Assistant Practitioners in the NHS: Factors Affecting Evolution and Development of the Role*. Skills for Health Expert Paper. Bristol, SfH.

Smith, M. K. (1996, 2005). 'Competence and Competencies,' The Encyclopaedia of Informal Education.' Retrieved 30 December 2011, from http://www.infed.org/biblio/b-comp.htm.

Smith, R. (1991). 'Where Is Wisdom? The Poverty of Medical Evidence.' *British Medical Journal* **303**: 789–790.

Sprinks, J. (2012). 'NMC Set to Gain New Powers in Review of Regulatory Framework.' *Nursing Standard* **26**(25): 5.

Staines, R. (17 March 2008). 'News Analysis: NMC Under Scrutiny.' Retrieved 11 March 2012.

Stein, L. (1967). 'The Doctor-Nurse Game.' *Archives of General Psychiatry* **16**: 699–703.

Strand, S. (2007). Minority Ethnic Pupils in the Longitudinal Study of Young People in England (LSYPE). Warwick, Centre for Educational Development Appraisal and Research, University of Warwick.

Strong, P. (1984). 'Viewpoint: The Academic Encirclement of Medicine?' *Sociology of Health & Illness* **6**(3): 339–358.

Strong, P. and J. Robinson (1990). *The NHS—Under New Management*. Milton Keynes, Open University Press.

Talbot, M. (2004). 'Monkey see, Monkey do: A Critique of the Competency Model in Graduate Medical Education.' *Medical Education* **38**: 587–592.

Thompson, M. (1997). 'Closing the Gap Between Nursing Research and Practice.' *Evidence Based Nursing* **1**(1): 7–8.

Timmermans, S. and M. Berg (2003). *The Gold Standard: The Challenge of Evidence-Based Medicine and Standardization in Health Care*. Philadelphia, Temple University Press.

Traynor, M. (1996). *Rhetoric and Rationality: A Deconstruction of Managerial and Nursing Discourse in the New NHS*, Nottingham.

Traynor, M. (2009). 'Indeterminacy and Technicality Revisited: How Medicine and Nursing Have Responded to the Evidence Based Movement.' *Sociology of Health & Illness* **31**(4): 494–507.

Tremblay, M. (1998). UKCC, Democracy and Accountability: A Review of 'The Regulation of Nurses, Midwives and Health Visitors', A Document Prepared by JM Consulting, Ltd. London, Tremblay Consulting.

Trinder, L. (2000). Introduction: The Context of Evidence-Based Practice. *Evidence-Based Practice: A Critical Appraisal*. L. Trinder and S. Reynolds (Eds). Oxford, Blackwell, 1–16.

UNICEF (2007). Gender Equality – The Big Picture.

United Kingdom Central Council for Nursing Midwifery and Health Visiting (1986). Project 2000: A New Preparation for Practice, UKCC.

Walby, S. and J. Greenwell (1994). *Medicine and Nursing. Professions in a Chang[...] Health Service*. London, Sage.

Walsh, M. and P. Ford (1989). *Nursing Rituals, Research and Rational Actions*. Oxford, Heinemann.

Wikipedia contributors (2011). 'Liberal Education.'

Willis, P. (2012). *Quality with Compassion: The Future of Nursing Education*. Report of the Willis Commission on Nursing Education. London, Royal College of Nursing, 55.

Wise, J. (2012). 'New Evidence of Worse Outcomes for Weekend Patients Reignites Call for Seven Day Hospital Services.' *BMJ* **344**: e892.

Young, R. (1992). The Idea of a Chrestomathic University. *Logomachia; The Conflict of the Faculties*. R. Rand. Licoln, University of Nebraska Press, 97–126.

Žižek, S. (2005). *Interrogating The Real*. London, Continuum.